Dr. Bob's

DRUGLESS GUIDE TO:

MENTAL
HEALTH

Dr.Bob's

DRUGLESS GUIDE TO:

MENTAL
HEALTH

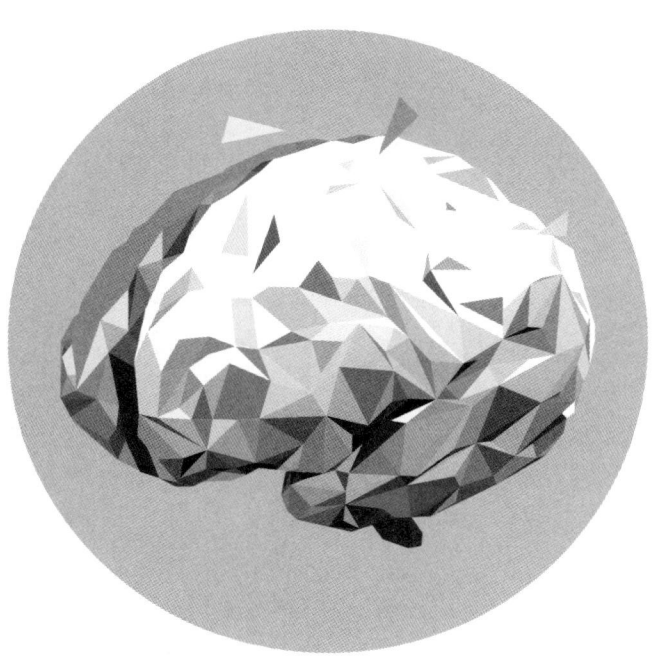

Dr. Robert DeMaria
The Drugless Doctor

Dr. Bob's Drugless Guide to Mental Health
by Robert DeMaria, D.C., N.H.D.

Published by: The Drugless Doctor
2001 Crocker Road, Suite 100
Westlake, Ohio 44145
Phone: (440) 471-7411
Fax: (440) 322-2502
E-Mail: drbob@druglessdrs.com
DruglessDoctor.com

ISBN: 978-09728907-9-3

Printed in the United States of America

DISCLAIMER: The information contained in *Dr. Bob's Drugless Guide to Mental Health,* is for general health information only and is not intended to be a substitute for professional med-ical advice, diagnosis or treatment.

The following pages do not create a physician-patient relationship and does not obligate Drugless Doctor, LLC to follow-up or contact readers of this book. In consideration for your use of and access to this book, you agree that in no event will Drugless Doctor, LLC, Dr. Rob-ert DeMaria, or any other party involved in creating, producing or delivering this book or any site linked to this book, be liable to you in any manner whatsoever for any decision made or action or non-action taken by you in reliance upon the information provided throughout.

Editorial services by Misti Moyer
Cover design by Ariel Vergez
Interior by Monica Thomas for TLC Book Design, www.TLCBookDesign.com
Interior Illustrations by Ariel Vergez

TABLE OF CONTENTS

INTRODUCTION

It has been my privilege to serve patients since 1978. I do not take it lightly that hundreds of thousands of individuals have made the decision to visit The Drugless Doctors in their pursuit of well-being.

Over the course of the new century, however, we have seen massive disruptions in terms of technology, such as the ways it has enhanced productivity and made our world smaller. It is almost impossible to wrap my brain around all that has advanced.

On the other hand, there are concrete health principles that do not change, which are not brought to the forefront of your attention until there is a pivot in the number of lives a certain health function is affecting. I stand on the health principles of your body being able to heal itself naturally, and since I am in the drugless healthcare field, I feel compelled to bring insight into one of those areas.

Today, we are in the center of a substantial mental health revolution, with an acute awareness of its grasp in our lives. It can be recognized in media of all types, oftentimes making a daily headline. Currently, almost every family I have a relationship with, or treat, has someone close to them who has trouble with mental distress of some sort.

These challenges can span from Alzheimer's to everyday stress that lead to mental fatigue and everything in between. It is so serious that most parents' number one concern I hear is: Will my child be able to survive in today's world? Seconded by: Will there be a drug addiction attributed to this? In different scenarios, this could, and sadly has, led to premature passing.

They are right to be concerned because with each form of mental health, the current path is to begin with some sort of medication, basically to see if this will "take the edge off."

In my opinion, it's obvious that this approach is not working for everyone. Do not get me wrong, there is a time and place for other measures, but first, let's look at another protocol with the outcome being a restoration to one's best self.

We all experience some sort of stress, or stress-related event often—for some of us, daily. Or, we forget something we should easily remember; or perhaps, we cannot focus on a topic long enough to pass a simple test. The approach I take for these occurrences helps alleviate the body signals caused by stress, which in itself becomes an issue, since most emotional or mental health challenges can be traced to stress as you will discover.

The intent for this book is that I believe I am still just getting started professionally, but with forty-plus years of experience behind me, I do have answers to a different approach. It's my duty to respond to what is happening in our society, and how, over time, with this unique insight, you too can have a brighter future. My view on life and my work is how I can help more people, and I feel this book is the answer you have been looking for.

My focus in this mental health book centers around the conditions and issues I have helped or have seen in my practice. There is a plethora of conditions I do not have experience with. I have not treated patients with post-traumatic stress disorder; my experience with schizophrenia is minimal but met with success; I have limited experience helping anxiety caused by sexual trauma or severe bipolar conditions. There are so many possibilities in the area of mental health it would be inappropriate to have you think I can treat them all. But, I can say if you follow my suggestions in the pages to follow you will, regardless of your current state of mental health, receive some positive experience since your whole mental, nervous, and emotional systems will have excellent fuel and function.

So, what has changed in the past twenty years to make this a more relevant topic today? My first thought is our addiction to media, in all its forms. Whether that is tracking who liked your last post or scrolling for the newest updates, we are all clinging to a screen at all hours of the day. When this happens, our brain becomes tired and carries an additional heaviness than there was before. Not to mention the mental fatigue from keeping up with it all.

Secondly, our food choices have changed, and don't worry, we will have further discussion on what a "healthy diet" for better brain health is later on, including a look at the combination of food and function. I would like to mention here that convenience has taken over homemade family dinners, where both healthy food and conversation do contribute positively to how we handle stress, which in turn impacts our brain health. Our family connections and the separation of core family values can be another element. The simple fact is that when the family is closer knit and regularly has open and non-judgmental conversations, there is peace, security, and an overall sense of ease.

Sadly, this is rarely the case in today's family life. With an increase in isolation from society and more technological conveniences, we find that humanity is at a crossroads.

One of these crossroads is the added stress and anxiety that has crept into our lives. These two are the most prevalent brain issues affecting someone coming into our practice. There is no difference between the age, gender, socioeconomic status, or location of these individuals—it affects everyone. My goal, in the time we have together, is to help you understand that there is hope. Together, we will examine what can be your solution and celebrate the freedom you will obtain once the pressure lifts.

This entire book is dedicated to assisting you when stressors (whatever they look like for you) overwhelm your own mental or physical capacity to handle them and to eliminate or suppress any break down physically, emotionally, mentally, or a combination of all three.

The following pages have the potential to create the confidence you desire to produce a healthy lifestyle and complete the journey with a happy brain. Let's begin!

Dr. Bob
The Drugless Doctor

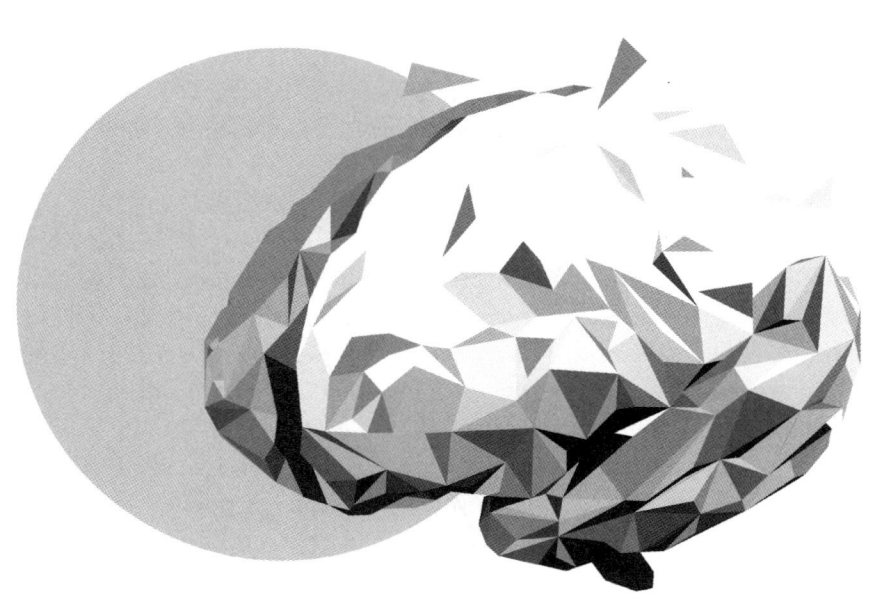

Chapter 1:

THE FUNDAMENTALS OF MENTAL HEALTH

Your mind is a beautiful creation and will be regarded as such in this opening chapter and throughout the rest of this book. We invite you to turn off all outside distractions so that you receive the foundational principles towards your journey to optimal mental health.

— Mental Note —

I could see my growing to-do list doing its best to get the better part of my emotions. As much as I wanted to, I knew that I just couldn't complete it today. Or tomorrow. Or the next day. My clarity felt off yet again, and my ability to focus, which I normally have, was all but gone. I struggled to outline not just my to-do list, but my entire day, that now seemed impossible to face.

Clarity, focus, and the feeling of being overwhelmed are all part of anyone's world, especially today. Their impact on someone with either mental fatigue or brain "overload" can not only be exhausting but lead to feelings of being unproductive or even disconnected.

If you feel this is you, read this chapter carefully to help bring things into proper perspective, and most importantly, give yourself a break. Everything is going to be OK.

Each day I am contacted by or have a conversation with an individual who is intrigued by the word, "drugless." They seem unable to comprehend how someone can be a drugless doctor, since they are bombarded with an enormous amount of advertisements sponsored by pharmaceutical companies.

This book is designed to provide you with a better understanding of what the drugless approach to mental health is, but before I do that, it is best to lay the foundation of how our society is evolving in this mental health space. When you say, "mental health," you are likely thinking about one of three specific areas: someone who has anxiety, depression, or memory challenges. I have so many patients who talk about living in a "fog" or do not recognize if they are coming or going, so they continue to live in a state of confusion.

A patient recently asked what could be done to get her off the medications she was on for depression. She has been divorced for some time, and the process of reentering the workforce was daunting. In another instance, I had a young man relocate from another city to the Cleveland area because he was distressed from a relationship breakdown. This move presented him with a new job (sometimes stressful in its own right) and persistent health challenges.

Both of these scenarios are an example of what is quite common in my daily dialogue with patients. At the end of the day, people want to be happy and loved. They come into our practice to recapture something they lost and desire the return of their health, happiness, and purpose for living. Many of the people we see have been plagued with mental stress of some sort for a long time.

> They come into our practice to recapture something they lost and desire the return of their health, happiness, and purpose for living.

I must applaud these two individuals, and the many more we have had the pleasure of helping, who desire to achieve restoration.

I am increasingly aware though that as a culture, individuals are becoming quite sensitive, or on the opposite extreme, quite calloused and polarized. We are also living in a time where many individuals do not take into consideration another's feelings and emotional health. If you happen to disagree with another's life perspectives, you risk losing a job, career, and even your relationships.

It is unfortunate we have come to this point of conscious anger. In my professional and educational experience, I have discovered that our emotions, whether happy or sad, can be traced to the function of our body. This right here is going to be the basis of the mental health protocol I focus on in this book.

> I have discovered that our emotions, whether happy or sad, can be traced to the function of our body.

Many people today have social anxiety because of watching, reading, or listening to the current events found in the news telecasts. If you already are contending with mental occurrences, it might be best to remove yourself from watching and reading on any screen—it is essentially the same cycle repeated over and over as you can see below.

The economy is always going to be in a continuous up and down cycle with highs and lows. Your favorite sports teams will be always in flux, celebrities will be in some sort of trouble, natural catastrophes—you get the idea. Yes, I have patients whose entire demeanor and personality is affected by news outlets. If this is you, it's time to get off this merry-go-round.

The reality is, our current affixation with social media and content overload is beyond the capacity of managing. I enjoy various types of media for minimal amounts a day, but I do believe our lives were easier before we started to like and share every moment. The best choice for some of you reading this is to remove yourself and participate in a digital detox. It's ok to have FOMO (fear of missing out) if it means you are giving yourself necessary self-care.

It's important to note our nervous systems, which include our emotions, respond to what is either real or perceived as real. Think about the last time you were at a movie theater right when the previews began, and the "roller coaster" would go up and down as the popcorn blasted right in front of you—my stomach still takes a bit of a dip as the coaster goes down the hill. Our world is becoming more perceived than real with virtual games, virtual events, and large television screens that transport us to another real or futuristic setting.

So, you may be asking: "Dr. Bob, why are we having so much mental distress and inward chaos in the realm of brain health?" There are many reasons for this occurrence. I've chosen to begin with the basics. Let's start by taking a look at food and function. Over the past few years, I have had the opportunity to visit many "natural food" expositions and conferences.

When I'm there, I see the vendors of multiple brands touting their products, hoping they will pick up distribution and be the next "big thing." However, there are even manufacturers of these "natural" food products that are using ingredients which can alter brain, nervous system, and gut function leading to more problems than they may take away. Since we rarely read labels, harmful ingredient changes often go unnoticed. This alone can sabotage optimal mental health. For example, agave is a common alternative sweetener, but it can disrupt the best intentions of reducing sugar, while the intake of its high fructose content can reduce insulin sensitivity and may worsen liver health.

> However, there are even manufacturers of these "natural" food products that are using ingredients which can alter brain, nervous system, and gut function.

The food manufacturer influencers say they are listening to the public regarding health concerns, but they tend to have their own agenda of producing products that are inexpensive to create, embrace a long shelf life, and appeal to those who have disposable income. This is the apex of the whole food challenge. They "control" us and our eating habits, until we proactively take a stand to stop eating their products.

Prior to the current digital age is when I discovered the role food contributes to our general health. My career gave me the opportunity to travel to seminars regionally, nationally, and globally. It was during this time that Debbie and I were able to visit many local health food stores. This is when health food stores were "health food stores." There would be incense of some sort arousing your sense of smell as soon as you walked in, and someone even might be drumming the bongos. I'm sure you can picture it well.

In these establishments, I loved browsing their book section. The authors of these books were often regional, with most of them self-published. Piecing together answers for tough questions was my driving force in discovering other's perspectives to help create new, innovative care plans for my patients. I enjoy continuing my research and education to better understand how to help my patients.

My curiosity led me to pursue a wide range of books, and then I discovered a paperback that displayed the metabolic "fat chart" illustration. The information there included the role of oils and how they impact function in the body. This was and still is the significant moment in my personal life and healthcare practice that opened my eyes and mind to the cause of most, if not all, health complications today.

Come with me now on a journey towards brain health. We'll begin with some of the basics I discovered years ago.

The Basics

First, there are a variety of oils found in nature. Some have names and functions based on the position of bonds or connections in the molecule. An example of one of these oils includes a family of oils called omega-3 (including DHA and EPA). It received its name based on the location of the bond at the third space in the chemical makeup. For the explanation of fats, I am going to discuss three oils: omega-3, omega-6, and trans fat (partially hydrogenated oil—an oil that is chemically altered).

The public has been inundated with the positioning of various oil names on front-panel packaging or the tiny print found in the ingredient list. Again, the role of food manufacturers has played a part because marketers have done their very best to control what they want us to perceive, or actually know, about fat—what is good or bad.

> Marketers have done their very best to control what they want us to perceive, or actually know, about fat—what is good or bad.

The educated and curious consumer of today can gain knowledge by investigating the role of fat function (and I do encourage everyone to be inquisitive). The access to documented information is indispensable for your personal, optimal health journey, and one of the reasons I am sure you are reading this book.

An interesting fact from the 1980's is that we have been told in the past that the "low fat," no butter diet is good. In actuality, it was misleading and contributed to mental health and cardiovascular problems, which still has its ramifications to this day. This low-fat, no-fat phase of the past, coupled with the present use of GMO oils and omega-6 oils, sabotaged optimal brain and nervous system fat production.

This is important because:

- GMO (Genetically Modified Organisms) grains are used to create the oils from seeds—tampered and sprayed with toxic substances including glyphosate, which has been found to be a cause of cancer.

> Omega-3 fats, from fish, flax, and walnuts, are commonly deficient in the average diet. When your body doesn't have enough omega-3 oils, it can literally become "on fire," since the oils reduce inflammation in your blood vessels, nerves, and brain tissues.

Understanding the role oils have on mental health is a significant key to your understanding how your brain and nervous system function. Our brains and nervous system tissues are made of fat, and you want quality oil in your body.

These two factors can interrupt the creation of the brain-friendly, long-chain fat **docosahexaenoic acid (DHA)**. When deficient in DHA, you may develop brain, emotional, or mental health challenges. If you want to achieve permanent healthy composure independent of medications, which are tricking your body, you will want to align yourself with the information I discuss regarding food selections for your new eating routine.

A good starting point would be to evaluate the foods you are currently choosing. Your principal objective is to focus on consuming omega-3 precursor food groups. Foods become the foundational building blocks used by your body to metabolize into the brain-healthy fat, DHA. Foods you could choose include Brussels sprouts, chia seeds, spirulina, hemp seeds, flax seeds, walnuts, green beans, wild caught salmon, cod liver oil, herring, oysters, sardines, anchovies, and eggs, which are laid from chickens who have been fed omega-3 flax seeds.

The best food choices I have found are those which do not have a label with ingredients typed on it. In other words, fresh, preferably organic, vegetables and protein would be your best option. Use organic olive oil (omega-9) for a salad dressing, alongside some homemade hummus and smashed avocado. I am not saying to avoid sunflower or safflower omega-6 oils, but limiting them would be helpful. When overconsumed as snack and packaged foods, these two oils tend to create a state of inflammation, which is comparable to your soft tissue being on fire.

> In other words, fresh, preferably organic, vegetables and protein would be your best option.

As we talk about the omega-3 foods and precursors, I want to help you modify what you are choosing to eat and why. Typically, and I have seen this most of my practice life, individuals as a whole eat for taste and comfort. Instead, I want to encourage you to eat for longevity. Pause for a second and ask yourself if the choices you are making are honestly going to sustain and support your current state of physical and mental health. This basic concept is the foundation which will safeguard you and create the mental awareness you desire.

Let me share with you an example of the harmful consequences of avoiding certain food groups. Apples help to thin bile, and not consuming them may result in gallbladder distress. There also can be collateral damage to your nervous system when one consumes processed and/or perceived "unhealthy foods." For example, refined grains, which have been processed with nutrients stripped from them, eventually rob the body of essential minerals and B vitamins, so they can't be used for the fuel your body needs.

Let's go back to gallbladder distress. Someone in my office recently had her gallbladder removed. One of the purposes of the gallbladder is to serve as a reservoir of bile and is analogous to the emulsifying dish detergent in your body. In my conversations with her, I mentioned that radishes are a food I would recommend for her to eat. These radishes would support the whole movement and thinning of bile by her liver. She looked at me with an unyielding look and said, "I don't like those." The reason she found herself in this position was she could not understand the vital role between food and function. It's true that you can get along without your gallbladder, but there are potential unfortunate consequences if you do. I have these conversations daily, and there are individuals who do not want to consider making any changes that would benefit their long-term wellness journey. Begin today and take a long look at how you can benefit by having an open mindset to new approaches.

> Begin today and take a long look at how you can benefit by having an open mindset to new approaches.

These foods I am suggesting are to help support optimal liver and gallbladder function and a healthy oil establishment. I am again adding the ever celebrated "Dr. Bob's ABC's," which daily consist of one-half of a red apple, one-third to one-half cup of beets (not beet juice, but the actual beet fiber), and one medium carrot, all of which I would recommend you buy organic. Patients always tell me how their personal health improved by adding the ABC's, including but not limited to, better bowel movements, clearer skin, and an overall feeling of being healthy.

One new letter I want to add to the mix is R. A radish is an edible root vegetable and helps promote optimal liver function. Had the patient I mentioned above added these few choices to her lifestyle, her health would probably be in a better state. I have learned how significant it is when one has a health condition that has deteriorated so much their gallbladder has to be removed. (You can read more in *Dr. Bob's Guide to Prevent Surgery* in the Gallbladder Chapter.)

The sibling to the omega-3 oil is the omega-6 fat group. This particular omega oil excels at supporting optimal blood vessel health, just like an omega-3 oil. The big difference is that food manufacturers add omega-6 oils, such as sunflower, safflower, and corn oils, in nearly every packaged and processed food item today. We, as a society, eat way too much omega-6 oils, because we perceive them to be a healthy and better food choice.

The final result is that omega-6 fats alter your body's function, instead of helping you reduce inflammation and protecting you like omega-3 fats. In a perfect world, omega-6 oils are excellent—they thin the blood and enhance the pliability of blood vessels. Too much omega-6 oil consumption causes the body to seek balance resulting in pain and inflammation.

Our bodies are magnificent works of art and through correct choices, have a means of creating balance in its systems. I have found much of this out through the analysis of thousands of blood chemistries. For example, one's LDL level may be elevated which suggests you may need more omega-3 oils. When one eats too many omega-6 oils, it is converted to a fat called arachidonic acid (see Chart #1 for the omega-6 fat chart and Chart #2 for the arachidonic acid pathway).

Omega-6 oils can be found in snack foods, dressings, or just about anything in our food system today via safflower or sunflower oils. Consuming too many of these foods can result in too many omega-6 oils in your system. Your body responds by thickening your blood, so you do not bleed to death from the potential blood thinning caused by the omega-6 oils.

Retracing how this occurred, food manufacturers steered away from the less popular trans-fat and soybean-based oils, which were placed on the "dirty dozen list" of foods we consume. They were keenly aware the public was avoiding trans fats, so they intentionally compensated freelance writers and popular "health" periodical editors to submit articles promoting the omega-6 fats as a "safe" substitute for trans fats. All the while, they didn't

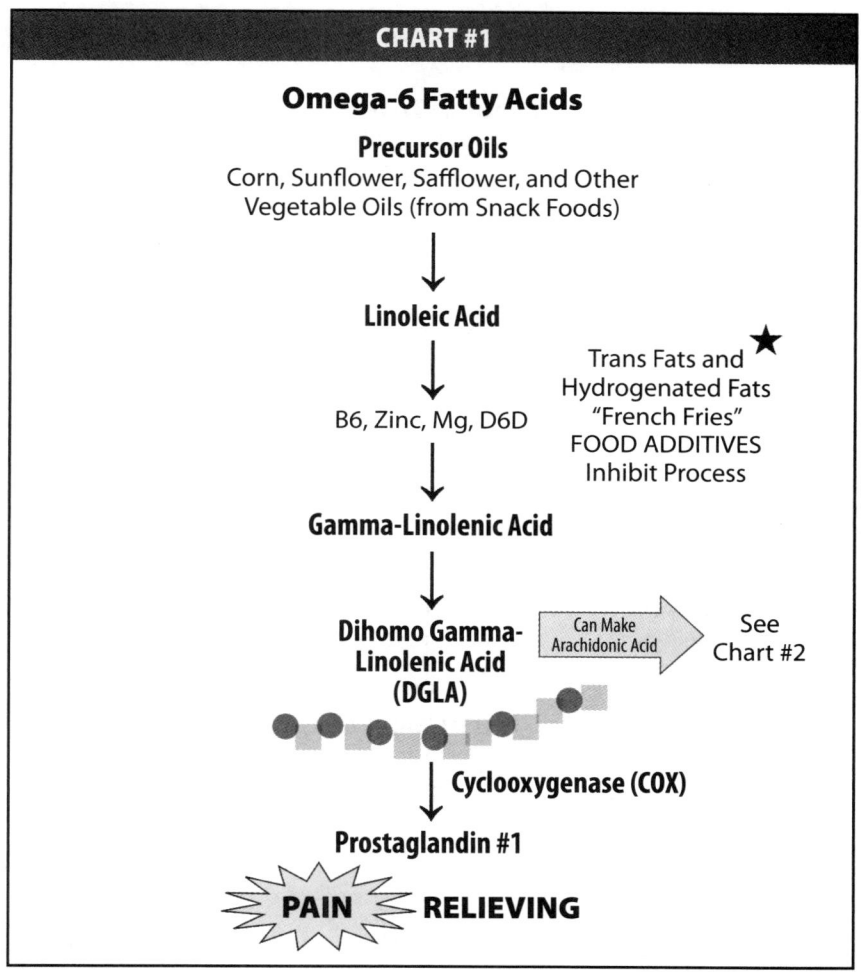

CHART #1

Omega-6 Fatty Acids

Precursor Oils
Corn, Sunflower, Safflower, and Other
Vegetable Oils (from Snack Foods)

↓

Linoleic Acid

↓

B6, Zinc, Mg, D6D

Trans Fats and ★
Hydrogenated Fats
"French Fries"
FOOD ADDITIVES
Inhibit Process

↓

Gamma-Linolenic Acid

↓

**Dihomo Gamma-
Linolenic Acid
(DGLA)**

Can Make
Arachidonic Acid → See
Chart #2

↓ **Cyclooxygenase (COX)**

Prostaglandin #1

PAIN RELIEVING

realize the new "healthy fats" were actually causing inflammation coupled with nervous system and mental health distress.

I am well aware that we have an abundance of omega-6 fats because of patient tests over the years. The fact is, most individuals eat inflammatory fats. We recently had someone experience a "brain bleed" from consuming omega-6 fats in excess. She was taking too many blood thinners, aspirin, and eating snacks filled with omega-6 oils. This caused her vascular system to have extremely thin blood. We advised her to avoid foods causing inflammation including sugar. She was recently

> The fact is, most individuals eat inflammatory fats.

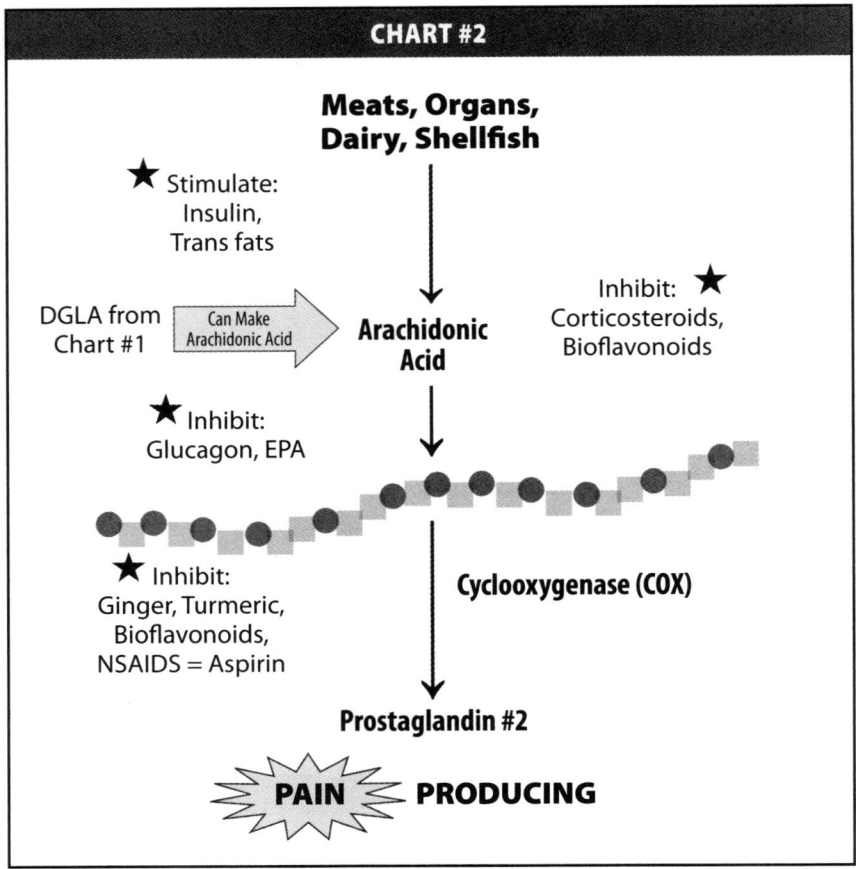

CHART #2

Meats, Organs, Dairy, Shellfish

★ Stimulate: Insulin, Trans fats

DGLA from Chart #1 → Can Make Arachidonic Acid → **Arachidonic Acid**

Inhibit: ★ Corticosteroids, Bioflavonoids

★ Inhibit: Glucagon, EPA

★ Inhibit: Ginger, Turmeric, Bioflavonoids, NSAIDS = Aspirin

Cyclooxygenase (COX)

Prostaglandin #2

PAIN PRODUCING

in the office without impairment and able to remember, navigate, and communicate without distress.

On the other hand, people who are on a low-fat diet, which was popular for many years, potentially can have what is called a **deep vein thrombosis**, or DVT, because their blood cells are sticking together in the blood vessels. I have seen this firsthand by those who come into the office who do not eat fat. Fat is needed to keep your blood vessels supple and prevent red blood cells from sticking together; otherwise, there is a greater risk for a stroke and/or reduced blood flow. There is a fine line balance: too little omega-3 or 6 oils can result in thick, slow-moving pasty blood and on the other hand, too much omega-6 oils can result in inflammation.

Omega-6 precursor foods and oils (safflower, sunflower, and corn) and omega-3 (flax seeds, walnuts, green beans, etc.) must undergo metabolic

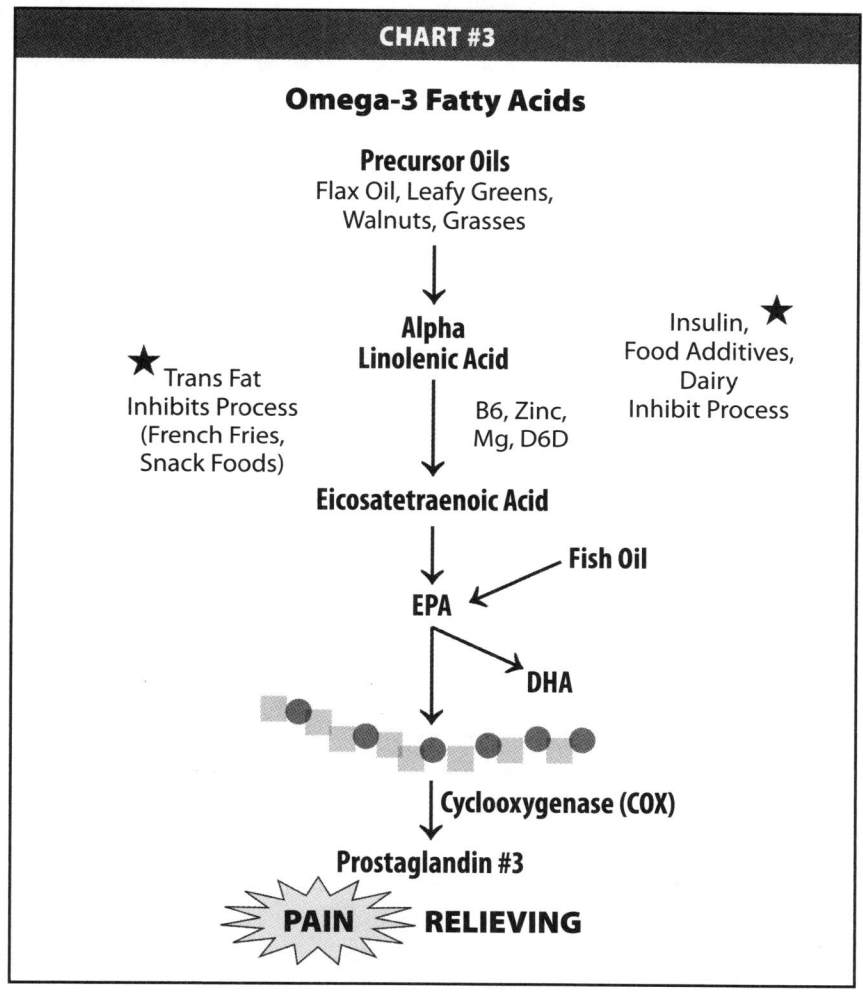

phases to be used by either the brain or nervous system. There has been a discussion by some individuals (those promoting fish oil) that the plant-based pathway for the production of omega-3 is not efficient, and in many cases, nonexistent or only 10% effective. I personally have found just the opposite. The plant-based omega-3 **metabolic pathway**, from my experience, is very useful when considered and supported accordingly. The real key to efficient long-chain fatty acid metabolism by the body is having enough "ingredients" or cofactors to complete the cycle to DHA and EPA. Simply put, you need the cofactors to create the long-chain fats as you would need the correct ingredients to create a recipe. All are dependent on each other.

Now, I would like to to direct your attention to the fat chart (see Chart #3). Take notice of the creation of the long-chain omega-3 fats: docosahexaenoic acid (DHA for the brain) and eicosapentaenoic acid (EPA for the heart). Also make a note of B6 (Vitamin B6), zinc, Mg (magnesium), and D6D. The B6, zinc, and magnesium are all recognized as cofactors, or support nutrients, required to complete the process of optimal brain fat. These three are deficient today in our food culture. The D6D, or **delta-6-desaturase**, is an enzyme, which becomes insufficient with age, and is part of fat creation in the body.

The good news for you and my patients is the fact that we can look at a simple blood test and evaluate if there is a deficiency in any of these three items. I traditionally use a serum blood evaluation plus the results of our physical examination, Health Assessment Questionnaire, and the consultation intake to assess cofactor deficiencies. Finding this out is imperative because we can make suggestions and create protocols to create a healthy state in your body, including the fats needed for excellent brain and nervous system health.

> The good news for you and my patients is the fact that we can look at a simple blood test and evaluate if there is a deficiency in any of these three items.

When looking at your blood work, for example, if the enzyme alkaline phosphatase is less than the optimal midline, you may have a zinc deficiency. Zinc is critically important for a portion of the memory part of your brain called the hippocampus. A zinc deficiency also causes the following body signals: white spots on the nails, memory loss, large pores on the face, slow healing of tissues, and blood sugar distress. Consuming sugar, wheat, and soy can deplete zinc.

If you suspect this, then a natural source of zinc would be to eat raw, roasted, or naturally salted pumpkin seeds. I must warn you to look at the oils used in the roasting process. This could alter your response if you use the incorrect oil. I do not feel that anyone should exclusively eat raw foods. In my observation, I would suggest varying every aspect of your diet. Consider raw broccoli. Its initial appearance is dull green, but when it is steamed or sautéed, it becomes vibrant. This displays that the fibers are broken down with the release of chlorophyll and become easier to digest.

There are enzymes with the abbreviation ALT and AST on a blood serum test, which are commonly low physiologically when an individual has a B6 deficiency. Vitamin B6 is frequently depleted with birth control pill use. This may be one reason certain females may have emotional and nervous system challenges. Excessive flax oil use can also deplete B6.

At our practice, we typically need to supplement B6 to get enough into one's system because it is commonly deficient and/or depleted. If you suffer from carpal tunnel syndrome, puffy skin and joints, ganglion (fluid accumulation on the back of the wrist), or a Baker's cyst (fluid accumulation located in the back of the knee), you may want to have these serum enzymes tested. These are common symptoms of **tenosynovitis**, or inflamed tendons. Some of the best sources of B6 include beans, poultry, fish, dark leafy greens, or a B6 supplement.

At our practice, we typically need to supplement B6 to get enough into one's system because it is commonly deficient and/or depleted.

DHA is the primary nervous system long-chain fat. This "friend" of our system is almost always deficient in those individuals diagnosed with any of the following: ADHD, depression, anxiety, nervous system challenges, memory issues, schizophrenia, dementia, or Alzheimer's.

Recently someone came to our practice for an assessment and their main health goal was for better mental health with answers based on objectives. He also wanted to be able to spend time with his children. His estranged wife had declared him mentally unstable and not safe to be around. The presiding judge granted her the restraining order, so he could not visit his children unless there was an attendant, and even then, it was not always guaranteed.

He was quite distraught when he first came into our practice. He was crippled with anxiety and depression. I suggested he complete a few weeks' worth of diet journaling so I could evaluate his eating habits. I also suggested we incorporate the Bloodspot Fatty Acid Profile (EFAs) or Omega Oils Serum Profile assessments. Both are amazing tools for detecting the levels of the very critical essential fats. The EFA Test can be completed in the comfort of your own home with a blood sample from a finger stick. The Omega Test is a full serum test requiring a venipuncture at a lab. (More information on each is in the Laboratory Testing Chapter.)

The assessment's sole purpose is to evaluate omega-3, omega-6, and arachidonic acid levels and the ratios of them to each other. Also, the long-chain fats, DHA and EPA, are assessed in comparison to each other.

The Omega Oils Serum Profile has been invaluable for discovering the exact makeup of the oil present in the patient's body. It has taken the guess-work out of creating a protocol and then tweaking it for the correct supplementation, which in turn saves time and finances while improving one's health results.

This test is also suitable for someone attempting to manage heart disease and prevent memory loss, depression, or anxiety. All of these conditions are serious and disrupting our society at epidemic proportions. (This has been happening since trans-fatty acids began to replace butter years ago).

So, let's get back to my patient. He completed the test and when he came to the office for his report, he was quite nervous. Much to his surprise, and not necessarily mine, his omega-6 oils were off the chart (they were as high as you could go in comparison to his omega-3 levels). The ratio was seven parts omega-6 to one part omega-3. In other words, he had omega-6 overload. His DHA, or brain oils, were deficient. The ratios should have been at least one-to-one, or at least midway in the laboratory's reference range.

I had some interesting conversations with him regarding his food journal. He would begin the week with a breakfast selection then draw a line for the rest of the week assuming I knew that he ate the same food for breakfast daily. He did not want to be bothered with the details of diet journaling, not realizing his food intake had everything to do with his mental state.

The eye-opening moment for him came when we went over his daily lunches. Each day he had a salad with dressing and chicken. Like I mentioned earlier in this chapter, the omega-6 precursor oils, such as sunflower and safflower oil, were deceptively labeled in the ingredients of his salad dressings. Sometimes the oils are literally and purposely clumped together with a statement along these lines: May contain safflower/sunflower/canola oil. The food manufacturers are quite savvy at masking the truth.

For his salad dressing, he used a popular "organic" brand but failed to look at the ingredients. He was not happy with me and had a few choice words (I'll let you guess what they were) when he found out he was pouring safflower oil on his salad every day. Over time, this seemingly safe and healthy ritual impacted his nervous system, not to mention his overall mental health.

I would be amiss if I said only the salad dressing's oil caused his problem, as our assessment showed he had other personal issues. But I am pleased to announce over time and with the correct diet modifications and supplementation, his oil levels improved. The legal team representing his wife agreed to have him evaluated, and he once again was permitted to spend time with his own children. This is an excellent example of how diet changes can impact function and one's life. The takeaway for your health is to read the labels. The fewer ingredients in your food, the better your health will be. Monitor your omega-6 oils if you do not want to have inflammation leading to your own mental challenges.

> The takeaway for your health is to read the labels. The fewer ingredients in your food, the better your health will be.

The sources for marine oil have changed over the years; you must make sure that the ones you choose are classified as safe and effective. In some circumstances, toxic oil can sabotage your best intentions if you unfortunately choose a "farm-raised" fish oil.[1]

Science Tampered Fats and Your Brain

Not all fats are created the same. When I was in graduate school in the 1970's, trans fat was just beginning to be promoted as safe because it was not on society's top ten worst food or dirty dozen lists. The heart health industry marketed trans fat as the cardiovascular savior. When this "savior" entered the food manufacturer's mainstream processing, it increased the shelf life of products. Trans-fat usage grew from being unknown to being found in everything. This occurred from the 1980's to the 2000's, when science realized it was an actual heart health villain.

Trans fat was perceived as a way of taking out high-fat cholesterol and butter for cooking, along with the elimination of lard and beef tallow. The oil producers combine vegetable oil (without cholesterol), heat it to extreme temperatures, and then add a few minerals and other compounds, while unknowingly twisting the vegetable fat oil molecule in the process. The alteration of the chemical model actually confuses the body at the cellular level.

There is a chemical term called the half-life, which is the time it takes a compound to be 50% less effective. Trans fat literally hangs around in the body interrupting fat metabolism function. Since the synthetic twisted trans-fat molecules cannot combine with our natural oil molecules, it causes a variety of health challenges in our bodies, including the nervous system. The half-life of a trans fat molecule when consumed as an ingredient in food is fifty-one days. Fifty-one days!!! (I want that to sink into your brain.)

The half-life of a trans fat molecule when consumed as an ingredient in food is fifty-one days.

The scientific community was delighted to promote cooking oils that did not contain saturated fat because they felt they had discovered a way to replace butter. They thought it would lower cholesterol levels, thus reducing heart risk. Little did they realize that margarine made with trans fat—labeled as partially hydrogenated oils—not only did not help our heart issues, it actually made one's heart health worse. Now with its use, the fat physiology caused inflammation of the blood vessels. With inflammation, all systems are affected, including the nervous system. Critically important information is transported over nerve coverings called the myelin sheath, which require a healthy layer of omega-3 long-chain fats.

Your body responds to excessive trans-fat consumption by creating more cholesterol, just the opposite of what science assumed. The body processes the additional cholesterol in a series of steps to make cortisol, which is likened to a firefighter using water to put out a fire. Cholesterol is not good or bad. But cholesterol is necessary for a variety of body functions. It has taken over thirty years for them to discover this, and many still do not know that fact today. The food companies succumbed to the public and the government's pressure in the early 2000's and mandated that all trans-fat products be labeled accordingly.

What is interesting about this government ruling is that a product with one-half gram of trans fat, or partially hydrogenated fat, per serving can be labeled "Trans-Fat Free" or "0g Trans Fat." Think about this point for a moment—when was the last time you or a friend ate just one cookie? (This labeling met the requirement to be labeled Trans-Fat Free.) I can almost guarantee that most people will eat two or more cookies with enough trans fat in them to alter their physiology and create havoc with their mental state.

A national potato chip brand challenged the public, "I bet you can't eat just one." And guess what, they were correct. The issue with trans fat is that it interrupts the creation of DHA for your nervous system. DHA is imperative for full mental health function.

When I wrote *Dr. Bob's Guide to Stop ADHD in 18 Days*, it is not about the fact that ADHD is cured in eighteen days. It is the actual physiological time it takes for your body to naturally "kick in" the correct mechanism for DHA creation in those labeled with ADHD, ADD, depression, and other fat-related conditions. Eighteen days is the half-life of healthy fat metabolism and why we saw participants improve in that time frame in the pilot study done for this book.

On the other hand, the half-life of trans fat is 51 days. You can understand why mental health problems can continuously linger. When you realize that it takes 102 days or more for your body to process trans fat, and if you are eating something like a pastry, cereal, snack food, or even salad dressing, there is a potential to never improve. Your body never gets out of the state of trying to process this fat, causing you to always be in an altered state.

> Your body never gets out of the state of trying to process this fat, causing you to always be in an altered state.

The trans-fat "empire" started to crumble in the early 2000's; more of the public and scientists became aware of the adverse side effects of this fat molecule mistake. Trans-fat consumption increased the amount of heart disease diagnoses. With the new labeling law, the amount of trans fat in the food chain decreased. We continually work in our practice to educate our patients and the public on the correlation between fat metabolism and brain health.

Cholesterol's Impact on Steroid Production

Cholesterol levels will naturally elevate as a defense mechanism to protect you. Sugar places a demand on the cortisol loop. Over time, if you do not have enough cortisol in your body, it will respond by producing more cholesterol for the steroid cascade to evolve.

You can see on the following chart, that cortisol is directly linked to cholesterol via the pregnenolone and progesterone loop. I have noticed when someone is under stress and their progesterone becomes deficient, it can result in other nervous system problems.

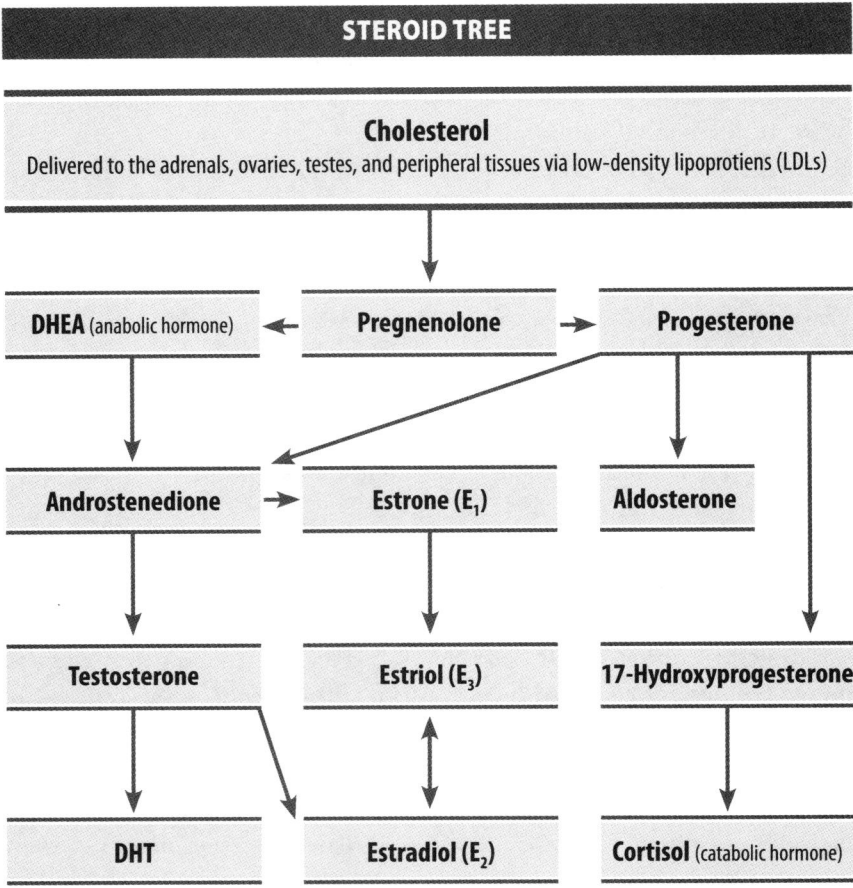

STEROID TREE

Cholesterol
Delivered to the adrenals, ovaries, testes, and peripheral tissues via low-density lipoprotiens (LDLs)

DHEA (anabolic hormone) ← **Pregnenolone** → **Progesterone**

Androstenedione → **Estrone (E$_1$)** | **Aldosterone**

Testosterone | **Estriol (E$_3$)** | **17-Hydroxyprogesterone**

DHT | **Estradiol (E$_2$)** | **Cortisol** (catabolic hormone)

Your nervous system is a diverse collection of sensitive, specialized cells, all of which are affected by food choices—this can go positively or negatively. The best part is, you get to decide. Now, let me share with you another case history.

One patient was diagnosed with multiple sclerosis fourteen years prior to coming to visit me, and I must say that she was in a bad state. She could barely talk and used a cane to walk. She also had given birth to several children.

During this time, she helped me increase my understanding of cellular function at the nervous system level. Because of my years of experience and the research I completed for *Dr. Bob's Guide to Stop ADHD in 18 Days*, I knew she was having nervous system challenges related to omega oil issues.

When a woman is carrying her baby as it develops in the uterus, the fetus places a demand on the liver. Your liver is the storehouse for many nutrients in addition to being one of the primary fat metabolizers in the body.

I have seen clinically that when a female patient has a history of miscarriages, they often have potential, over time, to develop multiple sclerosis, or other nervous system conditions. The nervous system is impacted because it is typically low in progesterone. Progesterone, as you discovered from the previous chart, balances estrogen or goes on to create more cortisol. When progesterone is deficient, it cannot be used as a building block for cortisol, which is necessary to manage inflammation. As you will continue to learn, inflammation is one of the foremost causes of nervous system challenges. Progesterone is also a necessary component for the conversion of T4, the inactive thyroid hormone, to the active version, T3. Thyroid dysfunction is also common with those who experience memory issues, depression, and those who live with stress.

Her Bloodspot EFA Test revealed she had little oil in her body. All of her levels were low, even the omega-6 group. The test also showed that she was deficient in zinc. As you will recall, zinc is a cofactor, or an important ingredient, used by the body to make the long-chain fat, DHA. To repeat, DHA is necessary for nervous system function and for the memory portion of the brain called the hippocampus.

The lab typically will suggest a protocol for us in order to return the patient to optimal function. In her case, she needed ten grams of omega-3 oils. This is a tremendous amount of oil for one person per day. Her nervous system engine was quite deficient, for sure, and her nervous system was essentially "locked" in position with no movement.

She needed oil, or her "engine" (nervous system) was going to blow. I suggested a protocol for her with a blend of omega-3 oils, and also liquid zinc and zinc tablets. Well, she responded in less than three months, and I am happy to say that she is doing very well and has had only one relapse after several years of drugless care.

This is an important point—her relapse occurred in August about a year after her "remission." She previously had an obsession for doughy bagels. She came into our practice not feeling well. I asked what was going on and had her fill out a diet journal for a few weeks. After reviewing her journal, I noticed bagels were written down every day because she thought since she was feeling better, she could go back to eating her beloved bagels.

It is not that bagels were not ok, but I am sure the gluten caused her intestinal villi to become clogged and sticky. She was not able to absorb and/or utilize the cofactors, especially zinc. Her body could not create the needed DHA for her nervous system. As a side note, I also supplemented her, as I do for all multiple sclerosis patients, with a liquid vitamin D emulsified product. (Personally, I do not promote bagels or anything with gluten, instead I promote a 90% grain-free diet.)

> Everyone's body can heal itself. You need to feed it the right nutrients based on facts and not a "guessing" game.

The moral of this story is quite simple: Everyone's body can heal itself. You need to feed it the right nutrients based on facts and not a "guessing" game. The response to most health challenges is right under one's nose—your mouth. This includes your mental/brain health. You need to be making the right choices for your body and not be misled by anyone who doesn't have the understanding of the correct health process.

We now have the ability through testing to evaluate the specific levels of each omega fat and arachidonic acid in the body. The significant breakthrough will benefit anyone who has mental, emotional, and/or memory challenges. If this is you, please consider completing the Omega Oils Serum Profile. The test was created to evaluate the role of fat and heart risk, and we have used it quite successfully to create protocols for our patient's optimal nervous system function and mental health.

Helpful Reminders

- If you have mental distress, I encourage you to begin with an Omega Oils Serum Profile to determine your omega fat levels. This test is critical in creating a health foundation. Your starting point would be to have a one-to-one ratio of omega-6 to omega-3 fats.

- Read all ingredient labels. Avoid foods with sunflower and safflower oils.

- Once you have your omega levels determined, follow the supplement program accordingly.

Helpful Reminders

- If your omega-6 fat, arachidonic acid, or linoleic acids are elevated, you may want to evaluate how often you visit restaurants. We are unaware of the fats used in other's food preparation.

- Consider having a serum blood metabolic test (Opti-Chem Profile) completed to help evaluate your cofactor mineral levels. The serum markers you are looking for include: ALT/AST for B6, GTTP for magnesium, and alkaline phosphatase for zinc levels.

- Avoid wheat, sugar, and soy products. These foods deplete zinc.

- Limit products with trans fat and/or partially hydrogenated oils. Do not eat packaged foods promoting "0 Grams of Trans Fat."

- Fill out a diet journal. What patterns do you see? How many whole foods are you choosing? How many times do you eat out per week? What is your beverage of choice? Are you drinking enough water? Water is important for red blood cell integrity; without enough water, red blood cells stick together transporting less oxygen to cells including brain tissues.

- Choose foods that will be used to make omega-3 fats, such as Brussels sprouts, chia seeds, spirulina, hemp seeds, walnuts, flax seeds, green beans, wild caught salmon, cod liver oil, herring, oysters, sardines, eggs from chickens fed flax seeds, and anchovies.

- Do you take an oil product? Is it an omega-3 oil? Choose an anchovy or sardine-sourced omega fat.

- Ladies, have you experienced a miscarriage? If yes, please complete an Adrenal Stress Index Test (Saliva). I have discovered those with low progesterone statistically have a potential to not carry a baby full term and/or are diagnosed with multiple sclerosis.

- Do you rotate foods? Rotate your food choices daily to avoid eating the same thing.

Chapter Glossary

All definitions were sourced from the *Merriam-Webster Dictionary* unless otherwise noted.

Deep vein thrombosis—A condition marked by the formation of a thrombus within a deep vein (as of the leg or pelvis) that may be asymptomatic or be accompanied by symptoms (such as swelling and pain) and that is potentially life-threatening if dislodgment of the thrombus results in a pulmonary embolism

Delta 6 desaturase—A desaturase enzyme that converts between types of fatty acids (termed 6 after omega-6 fatty acids), which are essential nutrients in the human body. (Wikipedia)

Docosahexaenoic acid—An omega-3 fatty acid found especially in fish of cold waters—abbreviation DHA

Metabolic pathway—The sequence of usually enzyme-catalyzed reactions by which one substance is converted into another

Tenosynovitis—Inflammation of a tendon sheath

Notes

(1) "Omega-3 Supplements," https://nccih.nih.gov/health/omega3/introduction.htm

Sources

Easton, M.D.L., D. Luszniak, and E. Von der Geest. 2002. "Preliminary examination of contaminant loadings in farmed salmon, wild salmon and commercial salmon feed." *Chemosphere* 46(7):1053-1074

For more information on the testing of marine oils: https://consumerreports.org/cro/magazine/2012/01/fish-oil-pills-vs-claims/index.htm.

Patient Testimonial

"I work in close proximity to The Drugless Doctors as an analyst. For about nine years prior, my concentration levels were low, my anxiety levels were high, and overall mental health could have been better. After listening to a presentation about mental health and how chiropractic care could help me from a member of The Drugless Doctors' team, I was willing to give it a shot.

Like I said, I was an analyst, and I would often sit at my desk doing work, but after a short amount of time, there would be a buildup of static, which affected my productivity. Since I started care under Dr. Bob's organization, I could tell a difference from my very first adjustment. I am doing better work, my wife is happier, I have more energy, I can concentrate, my mental health is back to where it should be, and lastly, my A1C is down.

If you are like me, and willing to do anything to help transform your mental health, give chiropractic and drugless care a try. Your brain will thank you."

– C.P.

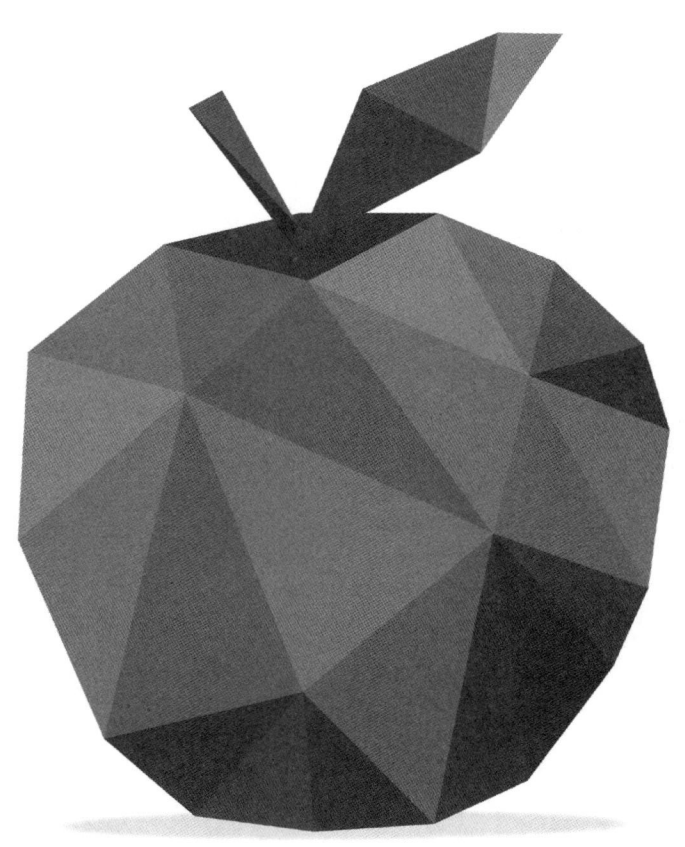

Chapter 2:

AN APPLE A DAY, HOLDS YOUR ANXIETY AT BAY: Food Selection & Organ Function

"Don't eat this," "Don't eat that," "If you eat five of these, then you'll feel ___," and the list can go on and on. It's no wonder why so many individuals might have some anxiety when trying their best to live a healthier life. The following few pages will go over these scenarios, plus how the foods you do eat can either help or deter you from a healthy state of mental clarity.

Traditional Chinese Medicine (TCM) was one of the elective courses I chose to take in the middle of my postgraduate training. Little did I know at that time, it would allow me to give you a blueprint all these years later to help you understand the principles of mental health. TCM assisted me in having a better understanding of the function of the body from an entirely different viewpoint. TCM's central healing philosophy is to provide a whole-body perspective instead of a compartmentalized body system viewed by the traditional Western "specialty" model of body performance. Studying TCM helped me connect nervous system function to spinal structure and its impact on mental health and emotions. As you'll see, mental health and body function *are* connected with your lifestyle choices, environmental surroundings, and food selections.

After receiving my Doctor of Chiropractic degree, I continued studies in advanced spinal mechanical function and whole-body orthopedics.

With continuing postgraduate training in nutrition, I obtained my Natural Health Doctor certification. The combined information helps me answer your nervous system and brain health questions. The correlation of food and its impact on spinal function holds a core foundation in my clinical practice.

I discovered early in my career that there is a physiological-altering role between trans fat (in this case, partially hydrogenated oils) and your nervous system. This revelation impacted the way I processed health questions and practiced in the late 1980's. During this time, I was able to piece together the association between pain and structural mechanics caused by an organ system overload and the role trans fat had on brain function. Multiple nervous system functions, including ADHD, depression, anxiety, and Alzheimer's, are all part of the fat, food, and function triangle.

Understanding how food impacts organ and glandular function is significant to overall body health. There is a looped cycle which means food is processed by specific glands. If the gland is overburdened, it can negatively impact the spinal segments associated with its nervous system function and cause the spine to misalign where the nerves leave the spinal cord to innervate or tell the organ or gland what to do. For example, when excessive fat overwhelms the liver-gallbladder mechanism, the vertebrae and nerves associated with that aspect of digestion via an electric circuit can overload. This can cause the vertebrae to move out of alignment. The cycle of eating and spinal function, which can impact the vertebrae spinal segment structure, is a full reflex that does, in fact, clinically impact one's emotions when observed full circle.

The process is analogous to the electricity in your house and the circuit breaker entwining together with, for example, the sensitive-to-the-touch bathroom and kitchen wall outlets. If an appliance is overheated causing too much electric demand (ex: when you overheat a hair dryer in the bathroom), it will not go back on unless you manually correct it. Now, let's look at it in terms of your health and well-being.

Food and Function

Initially, I was helping patients with traditional spinal care for the first ten years of my practice, mostly motor vehicle accidents and worker's compensation injuries. As time passed, I saw a variety of functional cases versus the typical neck and back pain caused by an injury. I observed my patients typically feeling great and happy. I also noticed at other times, for no apparent reason, there were those who were not so cheerful. I did not see a pattern caused by trauma or postural lopsidedness, as you would suspect with a structural, ligament, muscle, or joint malfunction.

Interestingly enough, as I was studying for a spinal engineering course, an instructor suggested to the class that the most challenging area in the spine to achieve pain-free results happened to be between the shoulders, or the mid-back and neck. What I am about to tell you solved the riddle, and it was life changing for me and for my patients.

I had a young professional come into the office with pain that felt like a knife was stabbing him, which he said came about without any injury, or anything else out of the ordinary. I began with my regimented routine that had worked many times before for those same individuals who may have inadvertently twisted their body from yard work, or other physical exercise.

The young man did not respond to the prescribed regimen and became disappointed, since he heard of the positive testimonials and wanted his "miracle," too. His discomfort was related to his food intake which impacted his spinal function. This led to pain. He probably ate something or consumed a beverage which created an agitation to the pancreas reflex pain pattern along his mid-back area.

I was putting together this sequence of events in order to help patients who were following a similar pattern. Patients who would come into the practice on Tuesday, Wednesday, Thursday, or Friday loved their care. Then there were some patients who I would see right before the weekend on Friday who felt great and would come back on Monday asking me what I did to them on Friday because they were in alleged "pain."

I explained to those patients who suggested this pattern, that I did not do anything different on Friday than I did throughout the week. At first, I was beside myself, but then, the metaphoric light bulb turned on, and my life was changed forever. My intuition led me back to my embryology class (from 1974!), where we were learning about the newborn developing in its mother's uterus. I looked at the book and noticed the pancreas embryologically originated in the upper back on the left side. Over the gestation period (amount of time inside the mother's uterus), it shifted to the front of the body where we traditionally understand the pancreas to be located: in the middle of the abdomen.

This led me to begin asking questions to my patients on Monday morning: "Hi _____, what did you do over the weekend?" The answer was typically: "I went to a wedding, ball game, movie, etc." My follow up question was now: "What did you eat?" The common response was: "Ice cream, cake, soda, candy, and alcohol." I knew I was onto something. Over time, I put the puzzle together that they were all eating some type of food which placed a demand on their pancreas. This, in turn, sent a trigger back to their neck and mid-back, or the original embryological location, causing PAIN. So literally, the pancreas' electrical connection in their mid-back and neck was impacted by a response from the pancreas, back to the spine, via the nervous system. I hope that you take the time to re-read this if necessary because this can save your life!

> The pancreas' electrical connection in their mid-back and neck was impacted by a response from the pancreas, back to the spine, via the nervous system.

Impact of an Overworked Pancreas

Most people think of the pancreas as the organ that produces insulin, but in actuality, it does so much more. For you, the foods and beverages you choose to consume can cause part of your mental health challenges because of the resulting excessive inflammation impacting your nerves.

I have a list of foods for you (which are part of an elimination protocol) that could cause pain and inflammation, including:

- **Pineapple**
- **Watermelon**
- **Dried fruits**
- **Raisins**
- **Grapes**

I have to chuckle here, because just this past week as I was writing this, I had two patients on the same day come to my practice with an OTC analgesic patch placed on their left mid-back region because of pain. When I asked them about what they did over the weekend...You guessed it; they ate sugar-filled morsels!

I know there are many of you reading this that either wear a patch personally, or know someone who does, to remedy pain symptoms. I am here to tell you the patch will not get to the answer of your pain. Many of you have been to doctors and have received therapy at different times, spending time and money without results. Your body's nervous system memory circuit remembers or still participates with the original nerve pattern thus causing the pain loop to continue.

The pain you are experiencing will not go away if it is caused by something you are consuming. I have seen cough drops, chewing gum, fruit juice, breath mints, "healthy" energy bars, and soda cause pain and inflammation—all with sugar in their ingredients list. You are experiencing this pain because you are eating too many processed foods. Your pancreas has to work overtime to keep up.

> The pain you are experiencing will not go way if it is caused by something you are consuming.

Taking this a step further, this process can snowball for years. Over time, I notice the vertebrae in the mid-back region will be reflexed in an abnormal position, with the spinal structural pattern being directly related to food—the model itself is consistent with those who eat a lot of sugar and drink excessive alcohol. The good news is it can be corrected with time. The overworked pancreas is trying to shut itself off, much like an overheated engine or hair dryer, which causes the circuit breaker in your residence to shut off when there is an electric demand. The scientific name for this pattern is visceral-somatic-patho-biomechanical-subluxation. Simply put, there is an organ-to-joint reflex, causing the vertebrae to misalign in an abnormal pattern.

The mechanism of food and function impacted one particular patient to the point she suffered with neck and mid-back pain for years; the pain was so intense and real to her that she was prescribed a medication in the benzodiazepine group, better known as Librium and Valium. Her case history and personal life has had a tremendous influence on my perception of emotions, mental health, and care protocols. She was advised by her mom when she was fifteen years old to make sure she ate yogurt for calcium, bananas for potassium, and whole grain cereal. She did exactly what her mom said and over time developed chronic neck pain that persisted for thirty years; that is when she came into the office. Those foods mentioned are loaded with sugar and placed a demand on her pancreas resulting in severe pain. The medications impacted her in a very negative way to the point she was married three times and in major depression when I met her. I had just discovered the correlation between food, function, and pain.

Within less than three months, her neck and mid-back pain was gone, she was able to get off the medications, and her life was headed in a totally positive pain-free direction. This is a very common scenario, and one of the reasons I wanted to write this book and get the information into the hands of people suffering without hope of a future and without the side effects of drugs.

The Impact of Toxins on the Nervous System

Your nervous system is the wire grid, which allows your entire body to work in unity with every cell. However, toxins from food, the environment, beverages, topical creams, or even the air you breathe can impact your cells. If you are having any long-term chronic health issue, especially nervous **anxiety**, depression, and "raw nerves," it would be very wise for you to begin documenting what you are choosing to eat and have a skilled practitioner evaluate the findings. Food journaling helps identify which foods could cause your distress, especially if you add symptoms you experience in the mix.

Adrenal Glands Significance

There is another area of significance I learned early on in my studies. There is a muscle-organ association with a pair of glands located on top of your kidneys called the **adrenal glands**. They impact every area of our lives and are commonly exhausted from stress, sugar, and fruit. There is a muscle that runs, or traverses, the front of the pelvis and attaches to the medial, or inside aspect, of the knee. It is called the Sartorius muscle. (Sometimes on a test question at healthcare provider schools, it is called the "tailor" muscle, since haberdashers cross their legs in such a fashion when they are sewing or mending fabric by hand.)

When your adrenal glands are "stressed," the associated Sartorius muscles physiologically weaken and the pelvis (which is composed of three large foundational bones in the lower abdomen supporting the spine) on the side

It is not uncommon for one of the pelvic bones to have shifted backward.

with muscle weakness shifts backward. As I am sure you are aware of by now, I observe bodies for a living. I can see the walking pattern, or gait, of a person and pretty much tell you what's going on in their body. The pelvic shift also shows up on the standing, or postural, digital films.

We notice when our patients are in the office for spinal corrective care, it is not uncommon for one of the pelvic bones to have shifted backward. These are the same patients who will come in with the statement to us: "I was not doing anything. I just bent over to pick up my sock, and my back went out." The back did not "go out" per se—the spinal function was altered because their adrenal glands were exhausted. They could have also just consumed a donut, bag of candy, or something which placed a demand on one of several adrenal hormones needed to reduce inflammation and/or secure ligaments.

Also, as a side note, take a moment and stop reading this book. Right now, look at your posture in the mirror. Is your left shoulder higher than your right? I'll bet you never observed yourself standing like you are at this very moment.

A simple way to test for your adrenal health is to have someone take your blood pressure sitting and record the number. Then, stand up and have your blood pressure taken again. In an ideal world, it should go up from a sit to a stand position. If your blood pressure drops, it's possible you may have a thiamin, or vitamin B1, deficiency. The B vitamins are essential for mental health and digestion. I hope you are beginning to see that one's mental health is one giant puzzle, with many pieces to put together in order for optimal brain function. You will discover the significance of the adrenal glands and depression in Chapter Five.

One last thought about food and function: I have noticed this for years—most of the people I see, either in the office or on the street, have a "puffy" look. Now, I want you to observe, in a non-invasive way, other's wrists and lower arms. Do you notice that they look "spongy?" Rarely do I see one's wrist bones. The body of the spongy or puffy individual is in a constant state of keeping all chemicals and potential toxins in a controlled neutral level. The body detoxification systems are holding onto fluid to protect itself from overload.

If your wrist is swollen or puffy, do you think your vital organs and brain are being squeezed? Yes, they are. Even your internal organs will not work as efficiently. You can easily do the "Squeeze the Wrist Test:" Take a moment and touch or feel the lower part of your arm or wrist area. You should feel skin, and then bone. If you feel fluid, you are probably inflamed, and it would be wise to avoid sugar, dairy, and gluten. You will see as time goes on, most of the modern day health challenges we face are directly related to inflammation.

> Most of the modern day health challenges we face are directly related to inflammation.

As you continue reading, you will see the relation of adrenal health and plaques on the brain, mineral absorption, whole-body toxicity, sleep pattern alteration, hormonal function, and a whole litany of potential brain and nervous system dysfunctions.

Helpful Reminders

- Do you have pain in your body? Is it in the mid-back region on the left? If yes, cut back on dairy, fruits (besides eating your one-half of a red apple), and sugar.

- Do you crave sugar? Sugar cravings can be reduced by adding chromium to your diet. I would suggest a Mineral Tissue Hair Analysis to evaluate mineral levels. Add a green salad to your lifestyle.

- Did you have your gallbladder removed? It would be wise to supplement with a source of bovine bile to support fat metabolism. Learn more in *Dr. Bob's Guide to Prevent Surgery*.

- Did you have films taken of your lower neck and upper mid-back? Look at the pattern of the small bones in the center of your vertebrae. Are they centered?

- Do you have a history of your back "going out?" If yes, have someone take your blood pressure sitting, then standing. Your blood pressure should go up when taken from a sit to stand position.

- Squeeze your lower arm and wrist. Do you feel fluid or skin and bone? If you do not feel skin and bone, and there is a layer of liquid, it is time to evaluate what foods and beverages you are consuming.

Chapter Glossary

All definitions were sourced from the *Merriam-Webster Dictionary* unless otherwise noted.

Adrenal Glands—Either of a pair of complex endocrine organs near the anterior medial border of the kidney consisting of a mesodermal cortex that produces glucocorticoid, mineralocorticoid, and androgenic hormones and an ectodermal medulla that produces epinephrine and norepinephrine

Anxiety—Apprehensive uneasiness or nervousness usually over an impending or anticipated ill

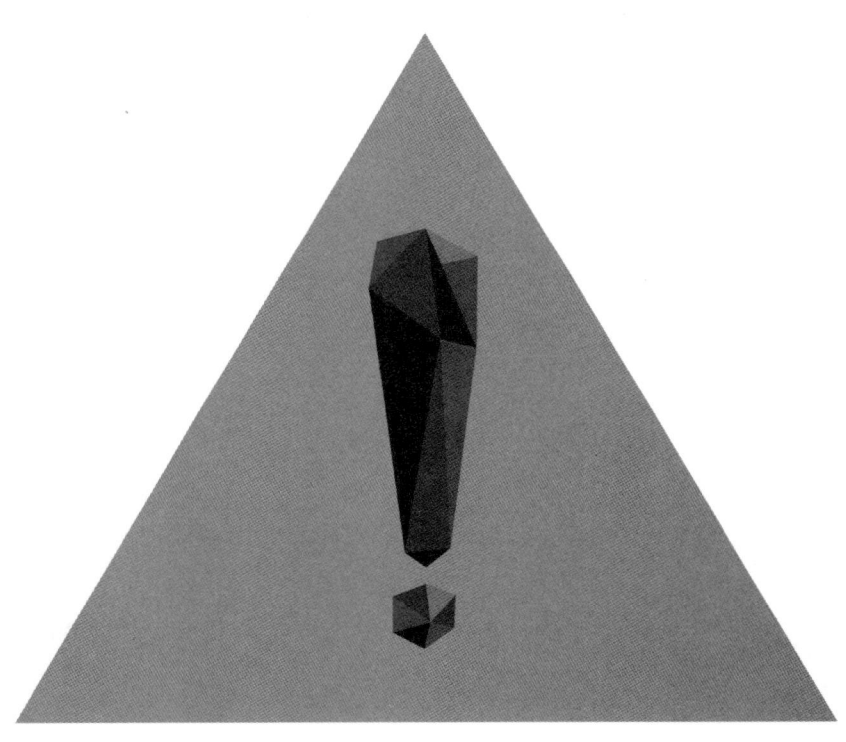

Chapter 3:

SIDE EFFECTS MAY INCLUDE

With every medicated pill you pop into your mouth, or inject into your veins, you may experience physical and emotional changes. Oftentimes, these effects may leave you in a condition that alters your quality of life. To regain control, read ahead and discover the steps to take which advocates a drugless approach to your mental health.

If you have read any of my other books, you know that I love talking about your adrenal glands. These small but vital glands are about the size of a walnut and are located on top of your kidneys, yet they have no direct connection with its function. Right now, I want you to think of your adrenal glands as your personal "First Aid Kit" and backup system for a vast number of hormonal functions.

Unfortunately, in today's society, the typical person is in constant go mode without taking time to properly rest. I have witnessed many individuals with mental stress, memory issues, and "brain fog" subconsciously rely on their adrenal glands even though they are already fatigued or near exhaustion. You can follow someone's pattern of exhaustion by looking at their stress levels usually combined with a large amount of sugar consumption. While sugar is perceived to relieve stress temporarily, it ultimately impacts one of the many chemicals, or hormones, that are secreted by the adrenals called glucocorticoid. This process, over time, can impair your memory.[1] Long-term levels of anxiety and stress placed on your adrenal glands can play a negative role in your ability to function mentally, resulting in unclear thinking and even brain fog. Raise your hands if I am talking about you!

Common Body Signals of Adrenal Fatigue (Exhaustion)

- **Weakness**
- **Dizziness**
- **Chronic fatigue**
- **Low blood pressure**
- **Weak, ridged nails**
- **Tendency to get hives**
- **Arthritic tendencies**
- **Bowel disorders**
- **Poor circulation**
- **Swollen ankles**
- **Crave salt/salty foods**
- **Brown spots, or bronzing of the skin**
- **Allergies**
- **Tendency to asthma**
- **Body weakness after a cold or flu**
- **Exhaustion—muscular and nervous system**
- **Respiratory disorders**
- **Bright light sensitivity**
- **Cry without reason**
- **Your back "goes out" for no reason**

One body signal I left out but want to discuss more in-depth here is an increase in perspiration or sweating. When someone visits our practice, whether it's their first or hundredth time, if they have a "film" of sweat on their skin, I can assume their adrenal glands are exhausted. The sympathetic nervous system response, which is the speed up part of adrenal gland function, creates a drier condition of one's skin surface. When your system is exhausted from poor food choices or stress, another system named the parasympathetic nervous system becomes dominant and sweating or perspiration increases. Personally, I believe that certain industries in America flourish (e.g. sunglasses and personal hygiene) because of an individual's exhausted adrenal glands. You see, many people wear sunglasses even on days when the weather is overcast because the sympathetic nervous system releases hormones to constrict the pupils. Even those of you who have excessive perspiration can associate it with adrenal fatigue. Women also need to get their rigid, chipped nails fixed. The adrenals assist in the regulation of mineral absorption, which is necessary for healthy nails.

Skin and Hair Conditions

Right now, I want you to come with me on a quick, or actually long, discovery road trip, that has lasted twenty years. This journey had one purpose in mind: to figure out when individuals were losing skin pigment, a condition called **vitiligo**. Upon first listening to patients, not only were they losing pigment, but they were also, as I engaged in conversation with them, stressed beyond belief, as if living with stress was their way of life.

Another body signal of extreme stress includes those of you who have lost hair in patches when under stress **(alopecia areata)**. If you lose all of your head hair, it is called **alopecia totalis**, while complete body hair loss would be **alopecia universalis**.

I scratched my head for years doing my best to determine what the relationship was between stress and the loss of skin pigment. Then one day, I happened to read an article about a comprehensive urine-based test and noticed the holy grail of information I was looking for. There is a breakdown product of **epinephrine** and **norepinephrine** (two of the many adrenal hormones) called **vanilmandelate** (VMA). Elevated levels of VMA in one's urine suggest a high turnover of adrenal hormones that are "fight" or "flight" neurotransmitters. So, if you are scared, in a threatening situation, or are stressed, your body uses these hormones up rapidly and frequently. There are two amino acids, or protein building blocks, called **phenylalanine** and **tyrosine**, which are the precursors for these adrenal hormones.

As the journey continues, tyrosine is an important factor here. Tyrosine and iodine work together to make thyroid hormone, and tyrosine is considered to be a natural antidepressant! So most of the time—notice I said "most"—patients without enough tyrosine may experience low or subpar thyroid function with one or more of the following body signals: cold hands, cold feet, depression, constipation, high cholesterol, morning headaches, fatigue, thinning hair, wide-spaced front teeth, and allergies from seasonal weather changes. Could this be you?

Now, this road trip gets even better. (I hope you made a good playlist!) Tyrosine is also a precursor for melanin which is used in skin pigmentation.

What I discovered was, patients who are extremely stressed and lose pigment can be depressed and have a subpar thyroid. I often do not see patients with pigment loss come into the practice just for that, but I have shared this with a number of them. One patient recently told me she had spent thousands of dollars on creams and lotions that have done nothing. I know what you are thinking, if you or someone you know has vitiligo—*can we reverse the process*? I have not used a protocol long enough, but I am sure that over time, it could be shifted. The process will require supplementation and lifestyle modification with a focus on less stress. The significance of this finding is: if someone desires to change their lifestyle pattern of stress and to stop losing pigment, we have the physiology to make it happen.

> What I discovered was, patients who are extremely stressed and lose pigment can be depressed and have a subpar thyroid.

If you or someone you know has lost pigment, I recommend first having your thyroid checked with a full assessment, and also consider the Organix™ Urine Test to evaluate your VMA levels which would suggest a need for tyrosine. VMA is a breakdown product of adrenal hormones with tyrosine acting as one of the building blocks for adrenaline. When someone has an abundance of VMA, it is logical to assume there will be a tyrosine deficiency. The Organix™ Urine Test, which is discussed in more detail in the Laboratory Tests Chapter, assesses the metabolites of whole-body function in one's urine. Residuals, when in excess, can determine what the system may be lacking.

As we end this road trip, we saved the best for last: tyrosine is a leading catalyst for adrenal hormones. When you are stressed, you are going to use up your tyrosine. When there is a tyrosine deficiency, you can potentially have low thyroid function with all the symptoms mentioned, including depression, adrenal fatigue, and when coupled with severe stress, the loss of skin pigmentation.

Additionally, as the process of adrenal fatigue or exhaustion escalates, the release of cortisol during the demand on your adrenals will cannibalize melatonin required for sleep (a quick reminder that the glucocorticoids impair memory). Individuals who have anxiety or depression, which can be linked with stress, have similar patterns, including sleep deprivation. That is why it is projected somewhere between fifty and seventy million

Americans are currently thought to suffer from sleep disorders and around 4% of adults use prescription medication to get a good night's rest, according to the Centers for Disease Control and Prevention (August 12, 2014).

Serotonin

In this next section, I want to discuss the physiology of serotonin, one of the chemical messengers, or neurotransmitters, that carry signals between brain cells. Serotonin is a neurotransmitter that controls or impacts function relating to mood, behavior, appetite, sleep, and bowel contractions. This is quite vital since all of the prescribed medications used for depression are doing what they can to keep your serotonin levels elevated.

As I shared with you about the VMA above, there is another breakdown product which I want you to know about called 5-HIA. The compound 5-HIA is measured as a marker of serotonin metabolism in the Organix™ Urine Test.

Many drugs, primarily antidepressants, may act in such a way that essential amino acids (building blocks used to create proteins) are lost due to increased metabolic activity to produce neurotransmitters. Elevated 5-HIA indicates higher than usual turnover of serotonin with potential depletion of tryptophan, which is used to make serotonin. 5-HTP can replace antidepressants, such as serotonin reuptake inhibitors (SSRIs)— Prozac, Zoloft, etc. Beyond treating depression, 5-HTP can also be used for individuals who have sleep problems or chronic pain, such as fibromyalgia. In my observation, 5-HTP should be the first option instead of the SSRIs.

There are steps you can follow to increase serotonin, including giving yourself more exposure to the sun. (It's interesting how people avoid the sun today or lather up with moisturizers that block the beneficial sun rays.) Another is to consume foods high in tryptophan, and one in particular, garbanzo beans[2] caught me by surprise. Tryptophan supplementation may increase the production of serotonin and excretion of 5-HIA. I would choose food groups with higher levels of tryptophan, including traditionally suggested items like turkey.

Serotonin production can be interrupted, or its output can be sabotaged by toxic substances like heavy metals found in our water supply, fish, and even the air we breathe. Pesticides (walking outside on the grass—an overlooked problem, even for golfers), recreational drug use, and some prescription drugs can cause permanent damage to the nerve cells that make serotonin and other neurotransmitters. Hormonal changes also cause low levels of serotonin and neurotransmitter imbalances. Lack of sunlight contributes to low serotonin levels because it is beneficial to get some sun (but not direct sunlight between 11am–2pm).

SSRIs

This statement is important for you to remember: SSRIs do not increase the production of serotonin—they negatively impact the reuptake. This can be a bit like "chasing one's own tail."

I briefly mentioned pesticides in a previous paragraph but wanted to come back to that here. For part of the year, I live in Florida, and I had a patient there explain to me that planes fly over certain areas at night, spraying the region to control insects. He said he is now notified prior to it happening, and they are advised to keep their windows closed. As I think about it, I rarely see mosquitoes, little worms, and other crawly-type bugs in Florida where I live. They are all but gone in my development. Another person in Florida shared that when he lived on a golf course, he used to get sick. He discovered that it had to do with the chemicals that were being applied, either as fertilizers, herbicides, or pesticides. Once he moved away from the golf course, his condition went away because his toxic exposure creating the health challenges was greatly reduced and/or removed.

> Unless you are being properly supervised by your prescribing physician or pharmacist, it is NOT wise to supplement with 5-HTP if you are taking SSRIs.

I would personally like to serve as your guide here. Unless you are being properly supervised by your prescribing physician or pharmacist, it is NOT wise to supplement with 5-HTP if you are taking SSRIs. You cannot just stop taking your meds without a proper plan, so you are going to want to work with your prescribing physician and a skilled natural partner.

Also, I want you to consider this option in case you are deciding on an antidepressant. I would suggest an Organix™ Urine Test and a Thyroid Panel prior to being medicated. This is a choice, but I would also consider an Omega Oils Serum Profile to determine your system's DHA level. I have successfully helped individuals navigate, minimize, and eliminate depression by creating a plan based on working with the test results from serum, urine, saliva, and hair testing.

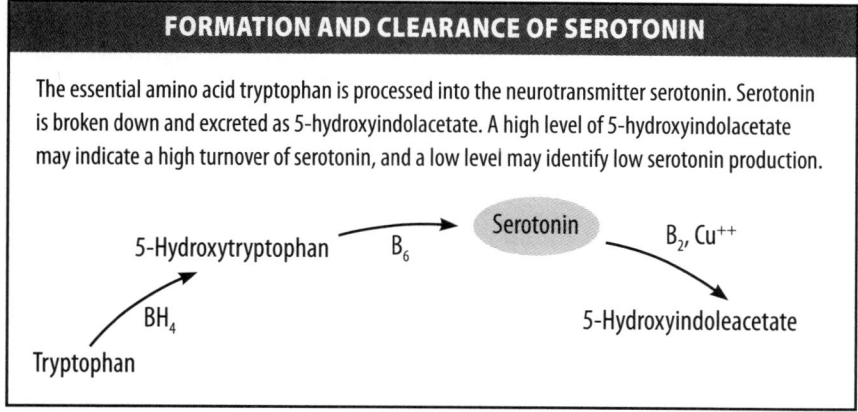

FORMATION AND CLEARANCE OF SEROTONIN

The essential amino acid tryptophan is processed into the neurotransmitter serotonin. Serotonin is broken down and excreted as 5-hydroxyindolacetate. A high level of 5-hydroxyindolacetate may indicate a high turnover of serotonin, and a low level may identify low serotonin production.

I am aware that up to 18% of the US population is on some sort of antidepressant. You will want to research how SSRIs improve your mood and what side effects they may cause.

At this time, it would be prudent to create the plan I outline for you later in this book. But here, I want to be totally honest: If you have stress and are cannibalizing your tyrosine, you are going to need to work on diminishing whatever is creating the tension in your life. You would more than likely be on the SSRIs for a long time. Yes, I understand sometimes eliminating stress is easier said than done. I would suggest an accountability partner to help point out ways you can reduce and/or alleviate stress.

Here, let's take a look at how the current medical model portrays SSRIs through the eyes of the Mayo Clinic. The Mayo Clinic suggests selective serotonin reuptake inhibitors are the most commonly prescribed antidepressants. They say the SSRIs can ease symptoms of moderate to severe depression; they are relatively safe according to their literature and typically cause fewer side effects than other types of antidepressants do. This is the medical model the massive pharmaceutical conglomerates want you to believe, but they do not tell you the entire story: once you are on them, from my perspective, your statistical chances to ever get off them are slim to none.

SSRIs work to ease depression by increasing levels of serotonin in the brain. The drug blocks the reabsorption (reuptake) of serotonin in the brain making more serotonin available. They are also called selective because they seem to affect serotonin but not other neurotransmitters. Lastly, SSRIs may be used to treat conditions other than depression, such as anxiety disorders.

The Food and Drug Administration has approved these SSRIs to treat depression:

- **Citalopram (Celexa)**
- **Escitalopram (Lexapro)**
- **Fluoxetine (Prozac)**
- **Paroxetine (Paxil, Pexeva)**
- **Sertraline (Zoloft)**
- **Vilazodone (Viibryd)**

I continually witness that once a patient is prescribed an antidepressant, they end up taking it for many years, even if they desire to only take it for a short time. On the other hand, when someone realizes they are falling into a depressive state, it's essential to focus on the cause of the depression, and from there, create a plan to help.

You must be aware of the possible side effects and cautions when using these. All SSRIs work similarly, and generally can cause similar side effects, though some people may not experience any (that they are aware of). Many side effects, according to the medical model, may go away after the first few weeks of treatment, while others may lead you and your prescribing doctor to try a different drug. If you can't tolerate one SSRI, you may be able to tolerate a different one, as SSRIs differ in chemical makeup; it is a prescribing drug "guessing" game, as it is with all medications.

SSRI Side Effects May Include:

- **Drowsiness**
- **Nervousness**
- **Agitation**
- **Restlessness**
- **Nausea**
- **Dizziness**
- **Dry mouth**
- **Headache**
- **Insomnia**
- **Blurred vision**
- **Diarrhea**

Sexual problems, such as reduced sexual desire, difficulty reaching orgasm, or inability to maintain an erection (erectile dysfunction—ED), can also be added to the list. One of the primary reasons patients come to see us when taking a prescribed medication is they want to get off the antidepressants because it interrupts sexual intimacy. A male may consider an

ED medication to obtain and sustain an erection. (Side note: nitric oxide is in the drugs used to manage ED, and it has been suggested it reduces vitamin B12 in the body used for emotional wellness and memory). An antidepressant can interrupt sexual performance, and then, when that is treated with medications, could lead to memory impairment.

Taking your medication with food, according to the directions, may reduce the risk of nausea. Also, as long as your medication doesn't keep you from sleeping, you can reduce the impact of nausea by taking it at bedtime.

> An antidepressant can interrupt sexual performance, and then, when that is treated with medications, could lead to memory impairment.

Which antidepressant is best for you depends on several issues, such as your symptoms and any other health conditions you may have. You will want to ask your prescribing doctor and pharmacist about the most common possible side effects for your specific SSRI, and read the patient medication guide that comes with the prescription.

They are generally described as safe for most people, according to the medical model. However, it has been said, they can cause problems in some circumstances. For example, high doses of Celexa (citalopram) may cause dangerous abnormal heart rhythms. Doses over 40 mg a day should be avoided, according to the FDA and the manufacturer. They also recommend a maximum dose of 20 mg for those over age sixty.

Other issues you will want to discuss with your doctor before you consider an SSRI include the possibility of different drug interactions. When taking an antidepressant, and any medication for that matter, you will want to inform your primary care provider about any other prescriptions or over-the-counter (OTC) medications you are taking to avoid drug interactions.

Antidepressants can cause severe reactions when combined with certain medications or herbal supplements, which can be very serious. You do not want to take any SSRI with 5-HTP, from a health food store clerk recommendation or Internet order. You would benefit more by working with a natural health doctor before you even get to the point of needing an SSRI.

Serotonin Syndrome

Let's look at an overload syndrome. It is possible that antidepressants can cause high levels of serotonin to accumulate in your body. Serotonin syndrome most often occurs when two medications that raise the level of serotonin are combined. These include antidepressants, specific pain or headache medications, and the herbal supplement St. John's Wort. Signs and symptoms of serotonin syndrome include anxiety, agitation, sweating, confusion, tremors, restlessness, lack of coordination, and a rapid heart rate. Seek immediate medical attention if you have any of these signs or symptoms.

For your own health awareness, there is a condition called **polypharmacy,** where a combination of medications can create a whole other set of challenges, including coma and seizures. I have many new patients who present to our practice prescribed other add-on medications, like Wellbutrin, which is an antidepressant medication that works in the brain. It is approved for the treatment of major depressive disorder (MDD), seasonal affective disorder (SAD), and to help people quit smoking.

Be mindful of any medications you may be taking if you are pregnant. Personally, I would have your thyroid level tested and do an Organix™ Urine Test before getting pregnant, if you are depressed. You will want to talk to your primary care doctor about the risks and benefits of using specific antidepressants. Some antidepressants may have an effect on and harm your baby if you take them during pregnancy, or while you're breastfeeding. If you're taking an antidepressant and you're considering getting pregnant, talk to your doctor about the possible risks.

> If you're taking an antidepressant and you're considering getting pregnant, talk to your doctor about the possible risks.

Suicide risks can occur with antidepressant use. According to the medical community, most antidepressants are supposedly safe, but the FDA requires that all antidepressants carry black box warnings, which is the most serious medication warning label. In some cases, children, teenagers, and young adults under twenty-five may have an increase in suicidal thoughts or behavior when taking antidepressants, especially in the first few weeks after starting or when the dose is changed.

I have patients in my clinical practice share with me that they have had suicidal thoughts. One went so far as to say that she was lying on the sofa in her house doing everything she could not to go into the kitchen to get a sharp knife and kill herself. This is serious, friends.

Anyone taking an antidepressant should be watched closely for any worsening depression or unusual behavior. If you or someone you know has suicidal thoughts when taking an anti-depressant, immediately contact your doctor or get emergency help. **(National Suicide Prevention Lifeline Call 1-800-273-8255 Available 24 hours every day)** Again, I stress that if you, or someone you know, is in that situation, consider having an Omega Oils Serum Profile done to check oil levels. Adding the appropriate omega oil or avoiding the omega-6 inflammatory version is a rational approach to help control optimal function without interfering with the SSRI.

> If you or someone you know has suicidal thoughts when taking an antidepressant, immediately contact your doctor or get emergency help.

Keep in mind, according to the medical model, antidepressants are more likely to reduce suicide risk in the long run by improving mood. SSRIs aren't considered addictive according to the medical community; however, stopping antidepressant treatment abruptly, or missing several doses, can cause withdrawal-like symptoms. This is sometimes called discontinuation syndrome. Work with your doctor to gradually and safely decrease your dose.

Withdrawal-like symptoms can include:

- **General feeling of uneasiness**
- **Lethargy**
- **Nausea**
- **Flu-like symptoms**
- **Dizziness**

Individuals may react differently to the same antidepressant. For example, a particular drug may work better, or not as well, for you than for another person, even in the same family. Or you may have more or fewer side effects from taking a specific antidepressant than someone else. If you are going to choose an antidepressant, your prescribing physician is supposed to take into account your symptoms, any health problems, other medications you take, and what has worked for you in the past.

Typically, it may take several weeks or longer before an antidepressant is fully effective and for initial side effects to ease. You may need to try several dose adjustments or different antidepressants before you find the right one. What amazes me about the prescription "guessing" game is you would be much further ahead by having your tyrosine levels, adrenal function, and omega oils checked before you embark on the SSRI journey. I discuss the half-life of oils in *Dr. Bob's Guide to Stop ADHD in 18 Days*. It takes eighteen days for the half-life of CIS oils to be incorporated into **fatty acid metabolism.** (A CIS oil is a natural fatty acid in which the carbon molecules lie on the same side of the double bond.) When we performed our pilot program with twenty-five participants for ADHD research, 80% of them responded remarkably well within the eighteen-day time frame. My goal is to offer you alternatives to the standard methods of treating mental distress, whichever kind you are experiencing.

> My goal is to offer you alternatives to the standard methods of treating mental distress, whichever kind you are experiencing.

Helpful Reminders

- If you are depressed and not on any medication, my suggestion is to have a Thyroid Panel, including TSH, T3, and T4, from your healthcare provider. Historically, I have noticed most primary care physicians only ask for a TSH. You want to see the entire picture. If your TSH is high, and your T4 is low, you may have a low thyroid and a potential need for tyrosine. If your T4 is normal and your T3 is low, or subpar, and you are stressed, you may need a protocol to support the conversion of T4 to T3.

- Regardless of whether you are on medication or not, if you are post-partum, you want to have the Omega Oils Serum Profile completed. If your omega-3 levels are low in comparison to omega-6 and your DHA level is low, you need to supplement accordingly. We use anchovy-sardine-based oil. Chronic, long-standing depression commonly begins in "unhealthy" mothers, especially after the second child. If you were contemplating having a second child and had any mental distress, you would be very wise to have your oil levels assessed.

Helpful Reminders

- If you are contemplating going on an antidepressant, you may consider having the Organix™ Urine Test to evaluate the metabolites created by your body function. This test will create a foundation to restore optimal health. You will be able to see if your system requires tyrosine.

- Have your blood pressure taken sitting down, and then repeat it standing up. This is a simple screen to evaluate adrenal health. Your blood pressure should go up ten to fifteen points with optimal adrenal performance. If you already have low blood pressure and are also stressed, you may consider an Adrenal Stress Index Test (saliva) to evaluate adrenal function. If your adrenals are exhausted, it would be prudent to assess your commitments and reduce them. Get to bed by 10 pm and significantly reduce sugar and fruit consumption.

- If you are currently taking an SSRI, I would suggest you slowly read this chapter again. Yes, it is possible to reduce your dependence on the medications. The Mayo Clinic said they are not "addictive," but they do create a psychological codependence. You would be wise to complete a Thyroid Panel, Omega Oils Serum Profile, and the Organix™ Urine Test to determine your levels, and then fix accordingly. I may suggest locating a skilled, experienced healthcare provider. You are more than welcome to visit us in Westlake, Ohio or Naples, Florida.

- Complete the B and G sheet (Chapter Five) to evaluate what type of vitamin B you may be deficient in.

Your Life is Important.

National Suicide Prevention Lifeline
Call 1-800-273-8255
Available 24 hours everyday

Chapter Glossary

All definitions were sourced from the *Merriam-Webster Dictionary* unless otherwise noted.

Alopecia areata—Sudden loss of hair especially of the scalp or face in circumscribed patches with little or no inflammation

Alopecia totalis—The complete and usually sudden loss of hair from the scalp

Alopecia universalis—The complete and usually sudden loss of hair from the scalp, face, and body

Epinephrine—A crystalline sympathomimetic hormone that is the principal blood-pressure raising hormone secreted by the medulla of the adrenal glands, is prepared from adrenal extracts or made synthetically, and is used medicinally especially to stimulate the heart during cardiac arrest and to treat life-threatening allergic reactions

Fatty Acid Metabolism—Consists of catabolic processes that generate energy, and anabolic processes that create biologically important molecules (triglycerides, phospholipids, second messengers, local hormones and ketone bodies). (Wikipedia)

Norepinephrine—A monoamine that is a neurotransmitter in postganglionic neurons of the sympathetic nervous system and in some parts of the central nervous system, is a vasopressor hormone of the adrenal medulla, and is a precursor of epinephrine in its major biosynthetic pathway

Parasympathetic nervous system—The part of the autonomic nervous system that contains chiefly cholinergic fibers, that tends to induce secretion, to increase the tone and contractility of smooth muscle, and to slow heart rate, and that consists of a cranial and a sacral part

Phenylalanine—An essential amino acid that is converted in the normal body to tyrosine

Polypharmacy—The practice of administering many different medicines especially concurrently for the treatment of a single disease

Selective Serotonin Reuptake Inhibitors—A selective serotonin reuptake inhibitor (SSRI) is one of the commonly prescribed drugs for treating depression.

SSRIs affect the chemicals that nerves in the brain use to send messages to one another. These chemical messengers, called neurotransmitters, are released by one nerve and taken up by other nerves. Neurotransmitters that are not taken up by other nerves are taken up by the same nerves that released them. This process is termed "reuptake." SSRIs work by inhibiting the reuptake of serotonin, an action which allows more serotonin to be available to be taken up by other nerves. (Medicine Net)

Chapter Glossary

Sympathetic nervous system—The part of the autonomic nervous system that contains chiefly adrenergic fibers and tends to depress secretion, decrease the tone and contractility of smooth muscle, and increase heart rate

Tyrosine—A phenolic amino acid that is a precursor of several important substances (such as epinephrine and melanin)

Vanilmandelate—A metabolite of epinephrine and norepinephrine (also known as adrenaline and noradrenaline) (Functional Nutrition Library)

Vitiligo—A skin disorder manifested by smooth white spots on various parts of the body

Notes

(1)   "The impact of stress and glucocorticoids on memory." *Clujul Med.* 2014; 87(1): 3–6. Published online Jan 30 2014. doi: 10.15386/cjm.2014.8872.871.at1cm2, PMCID: PMC4462413, PMID: 26527987, https://www.ncbi.nlm.nih.gov/pmc/articles/PMC4462413/.

(2)   Young, Simon N. "How to increase serotonin in the human brain without drugs." J Psychiatry Neurosci. Nov 2007; 32(6): 394–399. PMCID: PMC2077351. PMID: 18043762.

Sources

The Mayo Clinic link was also incorporated in some portion of the text: https://www.mayoclinic.org/diseases-conditions/depression/in-depth/ssris/art-20044825.

Patient Testimonial

"When my wife had a medical issue, I was nearing three hundred pounds and was under heavy amounts of stress, as you can imagine. One doctor, prior to coming to see Dr. Bob, encouraged me to take Zoloft. Even though I was apprehensive at first, because I did not want to be on any sort of drug, I listened to his recommendation. Within a short period of time, Zoloft was making me 'goofy,' which is not an effect you want to have when you're taking care of a loved one. I came to Dr. Bob seeking a drugless approach, and can now say that my prescribing physician has taken me off of Zoloft, which was the result of chiropractic care and a personalized wellness plan."

– J.T.

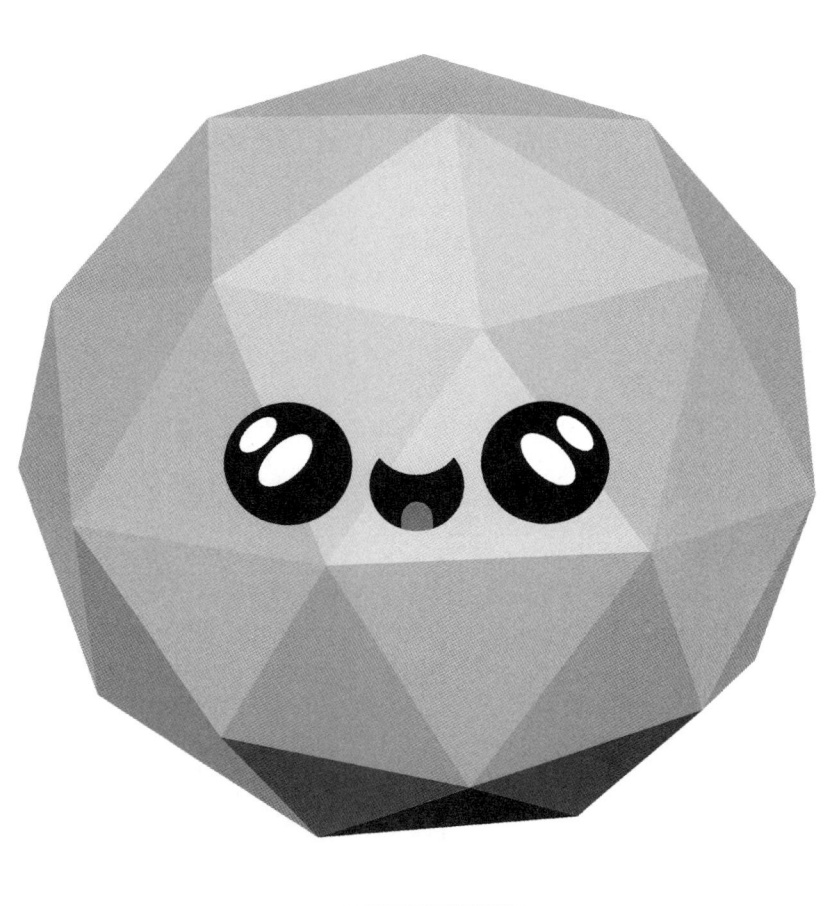

Chapter 4:

INSIDE OUT:
The Connection Between
Your Organs & Emotions

Not a day goes by when your body is not working around the clock, doing its best to keep you functioning at 100%. This is the case when you're happy, sad, stressed, lonely, hungry, and everything in-between. We're going to connect the dots in this chapter and demonstrate how certain emotions and organs in your body are linked, and your role to make sure they stay in harmony.

— Mental Note —

It was just a cookie on the floor. A broken cookie that my adolescent child dropped and didn't pick up. This time my emotions got the best of me. I'm glad no one was taking a video and posting it to social media when I snapped not only at them, but the entire family around the dinner table.

I knew I needed to find help, because these anger outbursts were becoming more frequent, but at the same, I didn't want to jeopardize my "clean cut" image at my company.

Could this be you? It may feel like you're holding onto a rope at the end of the cliff. There is an explanation and a remedy for you. The best thing is that it can be achieved naturally. Read on to find out more. There is hope for you today!

If you have ever watched *Inside Out*, the first line of the movie is, "Do you ever wonder what goes on in someone's brain?"

Of course you would say yes, as would I!

We live in a period of time where the central focus of individuals with health challenges is shifting their own perspective. Before, poor health was perceived to be based on a genetic flaw, or "prescription-drug" deficiency. For example, in the marketing world of dispensing both over-the-counter and prescription medications it is logical to think a headache is a body signal that you have an aspirin deficiency. Or, a pharmaceutical company will advertise, "Do you still have allergies? The current drug you are taking only helps manage three symptoms, while ours helps with six."

One correlation I have seen validated is when we actually discuss mental health in the context of having a happy brain and a properly functioning nervous system; it is more than just depression, anxiety, and Alzheimer's prevention. Optimal mental health also includes mental health challenges and emotions, such as anger, sadness, fear, and worry.

Anger

One of the first emotional glandular connections I discovered, and have witnessed firsthand with patients and the general public, was the association of the liver with anger. The liver is a complex and significant organ in the area of emotional and mental health stability. It clears toxins that can interrupt digestion which alters the absorption of vitamin and mineral cofactors needed for DHA brain fat function. The liver is an organ that contains and manages blood sugar, fat, and red blood cells, all of which are needed for optimal nervous system metabolism.

> The liver is a complex and significant organ in the area of emotional and mental health stability.

You also have likely participated in or witnessed "road rage," sometimes to the point where individuals can become quite physically aggressive in their driving and their gestures. This may lead individuals to record their driving activity with a dash camera just in case they need to share this information with the police or an insurance company in the future. Also, have you noticed how many people eat and drive? For me, I always see the drive-thru chains by my house filled, with new locations having TWO lines. The fast-food establishments even have advertisements with customers eating their meal while driving. I know if you have been on the highway for any length of time, you have noticed someone eating and driving erratically, and even shaking his or her fist at another driver because of some sort of inconvenience.

Most people don't know that the liver is required for optimal health and function. It neutralizes chemicals and preservatives you have touched and consumed from processed and chemically altered food containing toxic chemicals or ones that you may be sensitive to along with parasites. Also, with more individuals eating out or picking up a coffee to go, there are additional chemicals, toxic oils, and more found in these food items, which can create significant toxic challenges that tax your liver and can even cause liver disease.

I can see how one's liver reacts to the number of poor food choices because I treat many individuals today with large livers more so than at any time in my career. I now understand how your diet, beverage, and medication choices places a large demand on the clearing process of the liver. The liver combines proteins and sulfur to assist in detoxification.

We see fatty, enlarged livers on our digital, standing radiographic films. There is not a serum blood test which will consistently validate that someone does indeed have a fatty liver. A fatty liver is a physiologic (cell function) response, not necessarily a pathologic response with dead and dying hepatic (liver) cells.

This is a real concern of mine. Many physicians do a tap dance around the fact that food, which is the fuel for your body, impacts the function of glands and organs. I wonder about the comments being made in the special reports splashed in the media where food is discussed as medicine. I wonder where those in the scientific community have been? Do they not realize what kind of food we are consuming these days—processed and fast food?

Now, you may have a functionally enlarged liver, which is not in a state of "disease." Our organs respond to the demand being placed on them (ex: your heart can increase in size, prostate enlargement, kidneys create stones, bones adding or losing calcium). I like to ask questions when patients come into our practice, when they have quite the problematic history—this is just one way we are able to put together the pieces.

I have noticed over the years, those individuals who have extreme stress may also have anger issues. More often than not, their livers are larger than a normal-sized one. For example, the long and exhausting process of caring for a loved one who passes, significant financial stress ending in bankruptcy, or a hostile marriage breakup over time places an extra burden and demand on the liver.

When new patients decide to come into the office, often years after watching us on social media or by a direct referral, they are usually unhappy and display this to our staff. As we treat individuals and sort out and balance body function, they evolve into being happier. Some of the transition happens because they are choosing better foods; others may experience a total metamorphosis of body functions resulting from proper supplementation and/or spinal correction.

Prolonged liver stress can sabotage optimal wellness. You may not even realize your liver is in trouble because stress does not seem to impact typical liver enzymes. They are from poor diet choices, alcohol, prescriptions, or recreational drugs. I always look at our patient's liver size before their report, noting their results in comparison to what the normal should be. The liver should not extend past your lowest rib on the right side of your body. I am aware of those who have a history of gallbladder health issues, and/or its removal, may have larger livers. The gallbladder is the reservoir of bile located on the lower portion of the liver. A history of gallbladder surgery is a body signal of potential poor liver health.

The following are body signals of liver stress:

- Varicose veins
- Spider veins
- Increasing number of brown moles or spots (skin tags)
- Hemorrhoids
- Tender breasts
- Heavy menses
- Yellowing of the eyes
- Digestive distress two hours after eating, accompanied by bloating

The protocol we use for optimal liver health, first and foremost, calls for reducing dependency on alcohol. It would also be wise for you to set up a time with your prescribing physician to see what liver-impairing medications you may be on that can be reduced. Next, focus on eating non-starchy organic vegetables and cutting out any fruit consumption, which ultimately results in a non-alcoholic fatty liver.

Consider scheduling a time to meet a skilled healthcare provider knowledgeable in full body wellness that can help you create a protocol for liver wellness.

I'll end Anger with this, just like what came first, "the chicken or the egg,"—did the food choice cause the anger, or did the liver respond and the emotion of rage surface?

Sadness

One of the areas I noticed in the field of emotional health and glandular function is how many adults and children also have chronic lung problems, including asthma and bronchitis. They use inhalers as the treatment of choice, which of course is the standard protocol. Your lungs are emotionally associated with sadness and can be weakened with a severe episode or a constant barrage of unhappy news.

Your lungs are susceptible and impacted by stress. Stress of any kind places a demand on your adrenal glands, which rest on top of the kidneys. This pair of walnut-sized tissues have a variety of functions, one of which includes creating cortisone that reduces inflammation. The medulla portion produces adrenaline, which similarly helps manage lung function. People with chronic lung challenges are frequently prescribed lung spray medications with cortisone, which normally would be naturally produced by the adrenal glands when the lungs are healthy and not stressed.

Many years ago, my wife Debbie was having a chronic lung challenge with a cough and pain in her abdomen. I did everything in my power to help her. After several months of minimal and inconsistent improvement, I suggested she have an assessment with one of the massage therapists who worked at our practice. They shared with Debbie what she was experiencing was common during certain times of the year.

Our youngest son, who is now Dr. Anthony, was headed off to college. Like many parents, Debbie has a great relationship with our children. She was sorrowful and at the point of being "unhappy" with his departure from our home. (He was the "baby" you know!) Well, we treated the spinal segments associated with lung function and created a protocol to support her emotions with adrenal supplementation and specific oils, including **phosphatidylcholine**. This oil helps the liver-gallbladder function and is a building block for **acetylcholine**. This protocol helped her manage her lungs, mental distress, and seasonal affective disorder.

Today, I know patients are dealing with bullying, parental separation, economic stress, and social media distress. We are seeing more individuals of all ages with lung conditions. When someone is suffering from a chronic lung problem, I always ask what is going on in their lives. If they have a real or perceived emotional challenge, including depression (see Chapter Five), their lung issue is probably linked to their depression and/or sadness and is caused by something going on in their lives.

Body signals for severe lung conditions would require a chest X-ray to rule out a deep-seeded problem such as bronchitis, pneumonia, lung lesion, or other pathology. We also have our patient's blood chemistries assessed. The CBC (Complete Blood Count) with differential (see Chapter Eight) will tell us if someone may have a bacteria condition with an elevated **neutrophil** count and/or a viral challenge with a high **lymphocyte** count; walking pneumonia is typically viral while pneumonia with a fever and "productive" cough tends to be bacterial.

I treat more females who are carrying more personal and family responsibilities with many of them having chronically elevated lymphocytes, which strongly correlates to and suggests that they have a deep-seeded virus. I also have observed the white blood count levels, with a higher number indicating an acute or immediate problem and a lower count suggesting a long-term constant challenge. Either way, the numbers need to be addressed to create a protocol to manage the cell levels. I have a variety of supplemental tools we recommend based on analyzing the results of test numbers. So many times, I have patients come into the office who are taking a suggested, prescribed antibiotic. Yet, the patient's white blood count and other levels are within normal range, or the lymphocytes are elevated, which usually indicates a virus and antibiotics are not necessarily the primary treatment of choice. If this is the case, I also may suspect stress and/or food sensitivity as a cause of one's sadness and depression.

Here is somewhat of a side note: on the blood serum levels I mentioned along with the CBC with differential, I look at the carbon dioxide (C02) and chloride levels, which are impacted by impaired breathing. Those with an elevated globulin level (serum marker used to evaluate digestion) may not be absorbing the protein they need for their immune system. If someone has low serum mineral sodium with elevated potassium, they may have adrenal fatigue. The blood serum sodium levels may become deficient over time as the amount of stress one deals with can take time to create adrenal fatigue and then lab correlation follows.

I suggest a no sugar, no dairy, no citrus, no peanut butter, and no gluten diet for those suffering from sadness and lung body signals. All of these foods place a demand either on one's digestion and/or immune system function. I also cross reference and validate serum testing with a Mineral Tissue Hair Analysis, which is a type of forensic medicine mechanism at the cellular chemical level to determine areas of deficiencies or excesses. Frequently, I will notice high copper with low zinc, which suggests a diet that is high in gluten. Zinc is required for healing. We address all the findings and treat accordingly to reduce the impact sadness has on the lungs and entire system.

Joy

One of the most common emotions is joy, which is labeled in Traditional Chinese Medicine (TCM) as excitement, and even "over excitement." I have patients come into the office every day with some heart rhythm or strength issue or issues. Most of the ones with a heart concern I see tend to have anxiousness from some current or long-term circumstance, where they may not have had any control over the outcome.

The factors related to heart health vary with each individual. For example, the loss of someone with the subsequent realization that there is an emptiness or void, possibly results in heart distress, especially if there is not a short-term positive resolve.

The heart industry, and I say this with all due respect, is big business for the established, large, medical institutions, and is impacted by the emotional state of the public.

I have had patients receive a device that electronically supports their heart rhythm, such as a pacemaker, which positively changes their lives immediately. I also have patients respond to spinal correction when applied to the upper mid-back and lower neck area—the area where cranial and other nerves pass through on the way to tell the heart what to do.

Hardship and grief from the loss of a loved one can result in anxiety. I have patients consistently tell me their heart palpitations have gone away with either spinal correction, which impacts the nervous system, dietary changes, or a combination of both. The consumption of sugar affects heart function because it depletes mineral and other cofactors required to make the long-chain fatty acids necessary for heart integrity. Sugar consumption also depletes B vitamins that are necessary for the heart muscle to close heart valves in a timely fashion.

We use a tool in our practice called a Heart Sound Recorder, or HSR, which can digitally take the vibrational sound created by the heart valve opening and closing and record the sounds as a digital graph on a computer screen. The heart sounds can be quite long when a vitamin B deficiency is present. I have noticed erratic heart valve closure when someone eats wheat. Gluten in the diet literally "glues" the small villi or projections together which are found in the outer layers of the intestinal lining. The gluing of the villi prevents the absorption of vitamin and minerals impacting heart function.

Your heart is also responsible for moving fluids throughout your body. When the heart is tired or distressed, most commonly from stress or poor food choices, one can see how someone can become impatient. Much of the medication prescribed today focusing on heart health is designed to manage cholesterol, which is not necessarily the universal answer. Cholesterol is the basic building block for steroids in the body: testosterone, estrogen, progesterone, cortisol, aldosterone, and others.

A rough rule of thumb here: when your total cholesterol is elevated with normal **HDL**, also called the "good" one by some (what I call exercise cholesterol), and the **LDL** levels are elevated, where the medical model says "bad," you likely have inflammation and need heart and brain-healthy omega-3 oils. This is what I have discovered and want to pass on to you. If your cholesterol is elevated and your triglycerides (blood fat) is normal, then you have stress. If, on the other hand, your cholesterol is elevated and your triglycerides are elevated, then you are probably eating too many refined grains and sugar. Stress, real or perceived, places a demand on your body to make more cholesterol, which in turn continues to make hormones that support the "steroid tree." (For reference see the Steroid Tree on page 18.)

If your cholesterol and triglycerides are elevated, you more than likely have your hand in the "cookie jar." Sugar and stress will raise cholesterol. Stress definitely impacts heart function, and it will also create a desire for salty foods. So, you can see there is a correlation between the heart, emotions, stress, and energy.

Cholesterol Up & Triglycerides Normal = Stress

Cholesterol Up & Triglycerides Elevated = Diet Distress (Sugar & Trans Fat)

I also want to share what I fondly call the "Working Woman Syndrome." This lady is usually over age fifty managing her career, aging parents, adult children, spouse, grandchildren, and possibly stepchildren and step-grandchildren. These ladies come into the office with anxiety, stress, and heart palpitations, along with high blood pressure and constipation. We commonly support this with magnesium. Now just because you read this does not mean I am suggesting your challenge will be alleviated by taking a magnesium pill. There are a lot of different types of magnesium, and we test our patients to determine which one is best for them.

Worry

The spleen is a gland that is not discussed very often unless you have had the misfortune of being in a motor vehicle accident and it was severely damaged and needed to be removed. Your spleen is located in the left quadrant of your abdomen. It is a unique gland, since it plays a major role in your immune system and the management of red blood cells.

Interestingly enough, the TCM association with the spleen encompasses both worry and anxiety; they work hand in hand with each other. Most people, from my perspective, who tend to have anxiety, also tend to worry a lot. We have been able to help many "worriers" by adding the correct B vitamins and minerals for them to have better mental capabilities.

Most people do not consciously think about their immune system. People who worry tend to always be "sick" or have something "wrong." Back when I was an undergrad student, I used to work in a lumber yard. The wife of the gentleman who I worked for was what you would call a "worry wart." She was always sick, I mean, always. I have patients in the office that are always worrying about everything, and guess what? They too are always sick.

> People who worry tend to always be "sick" or have something "wrong."

What is interesting, is when I evaluate patients through a variety of Bio-Feedback and other electronic tools, the spleen shows up with those who tend to have **dysbiosis** or unfriendly organism growth in their systems. I also see the spleen as a marker when people tend to eat food that compromises their immune system.

If we have a patient come into the office and their red blood cells are not exactly right, or spot on, we will support the spleen with neonatal glandular bovine or porcine nucleoproteins. Over time, we will see improvement in one's red blood cell count.

Recently, a young woman came to our practice with severe mental stress; her mom explained that she suffered from a "personality" disorder. She had anxiety for years, a poor self-image, and did not have a concrete plan for her future. Her stress could have stemmed from first, ending a four-year relationship with someone; second, her parents were divorced; third, she had a new stepfather; and fourth, she had a new stepsibling. When I spoke with her, she was pleasant, but became very agitated when I asked about what her goals were in life. I recommended the Bio-Feedback Electronic Test, which is an objective measurement via a galvanic skin response specifically for her case. The test results suggested a spleen protocol that validated her presenting symptoms and glandular correlation. I associated the spleen with her anxiety, worry, and a weak immune system.

Work Skill Sets

I like to visit local farmer's markets, and on my last trip something happened that gave me a new revelation on skill sets in a work environment. The attendant at the booth I was purchasing from was doing an excellent job tallying all the fresh produce in her head without a calculator. She looked at me and said, "My sister could not do this. She has performance anxiety." She proceeded to calculate the charges, took the money for the transaction, and gave me change. I pondered how many people who are not in the right role appear to have major emotional issues.

> Some of the anxiety people experience is based on them being in the wrong position because they may not have the skill sets needed for that job.

At our practice we have employed a variety of well-qualified, or what appeared to be well-qualified personnel during the interview process, only to see them meltdown when they were in the office working with patients and completing tasks. Within a week I could see they were not skilled enough for the position they were hired for. Now, these are all well-intentioned individuals, but I also want to point out, some of the anxiety people experience is based on them being in the wrong position because they may not have the skill sets needed for that job.

As for me, I am not strong in math and I would kindly decline an invitation to be in a professional position in that realm. I am not saying I could not learn the necessary skills in mathematics; it is just not my strong suit. I want to make a point here: if you have anxiety in your marriage, job, neighborhood, or whatever it is, maybe you are not prepared, and either need to walk away, seek counseling, and/or obtain the necessary skills. I am aware that social media has placed this unrealistic demand on our desire to be the best and to have it all without any consequences—just like the young lady who became agitated with me. Yes, it is possible that she has a chemical imbalance, and yes, she was placed in an awkward environment with her family and school training, but she also had added stress from her home environment. She had to realize that something on her end needed to change.

I have a large number of men come into the practice, usually between the ages of thirty-five and forty-five. They often say the same thing: "I am on Zoloft." Most, if not all have anxiety, some of which I see is from their job, financial pressures, and other personal demands. My kind answer to them is always: your earning power will never equal your yearning power. There will always be something newer, faster, and better. They want to take the edge off, and there are healthier ways to deal with brain/mental health as you are discovering.

Helpful Reminders

- Schedule lumbar pelvis films with your natural physician, or skilled chiropractor, and have the size of your liver assessed. Evaluate the body signals discussed: varicose veins, spider veins, skin tags, hemorrhoids, tender breasts, heavy menses, yellowing of the eyes, and digestive distress occurring two hours after eating with bloating. If you have more than five, you may have an organ, which is functionally stressed, impacting your emotional state.

- If you have a chronic lung challenge, have a CBC with differential completed and have the numbers analyzed and then supplement and/or make lifestyle changes accordingly. Neutrophils tend to be elevated with a bacterial issue, while lymphocytes increase with a viral challenge. Depending on your results, you will want to address the source of sadness and/or depression.

Helpful Re*mind*ers

- Locate an experienced healthcare provider who can monitor heart sound function with an electronic stethoscope. Follow the patterns and treat accordingly.

- Consider an Adrenal Stress Index Test (saliva test) or a blood serum assessment to evaluate your sodium and potassium levels. We create protocols to support adrenal function; remember stress sabotages adrenal health. Optimal adrenal health supports optimal mental health.

- Look at the CBC with differential and check how your levels are doing. If there appears to be areas of high and low without a pattern, it is possible your spleen requires assistance.

- Look at your total cholesterol. Is it above 225? Are your triglycerides within the normal range? If your triglycerides are within normal with an elevated total cholesterol, I can assure you, there is stress in your life.

- Are you happy where you are at in life? If not, what can be logically modified to improve your self-image and self-talk? What action steps can you take to improve your perception of reality?

Chapter Glossary

All definitions were sourced from the *Merriam-Webster Dictionary* unless otherwise noted.

Acetylcholine—A neurotransmitter released at autonomic synapses and neuromuscular junctions and formed enzymatically in the tissues from choline

Dysbiosis—A microbial imbalance or maladaptation on or inside the body, such as an impaired microbiota. (Wikipedia)

HDL Cholesterol—A lipoprotein of blood plasma that is composed of a high proportion of protein with little triglyceride and cholesterol and that is correlated with reduced risk of atherosclerosis.

LDL Cholesterol—A lipoprotein of blood plasma that is composed of a moderate proportion of protein with little triglyceride and a high proportion of cholesterol and that is associated with increased probability of developing atherosclerosis.

Lymphocyte—any of the colorless weakly motile cells originating from stem cells and differentiating in lymphoid tissue (as of the thymus or bone marrow) that are the typical cellular elements of lymph, include the cellular mediators of immunity, and constitute 20 to 30 percent of the white blood cells of normal human blood

Phosphatidylcholine—Phosphatidylcholine (PC) is a phospholipid attached to a choline particle. Phospholipids contain fatty acids, glycerol, and phosphorous.

The phosphorous part of the phospholipid substance — the lecithin — is made up of PC. For this reason, the terms phosphatidylcholine and lecithin are often used interchangeably, although they're different. Foods that contain lecithin are the best dietary sources of PC. (Healthline—https://www.healthline.com/health/food-nutrition/phosphatidylcholine)

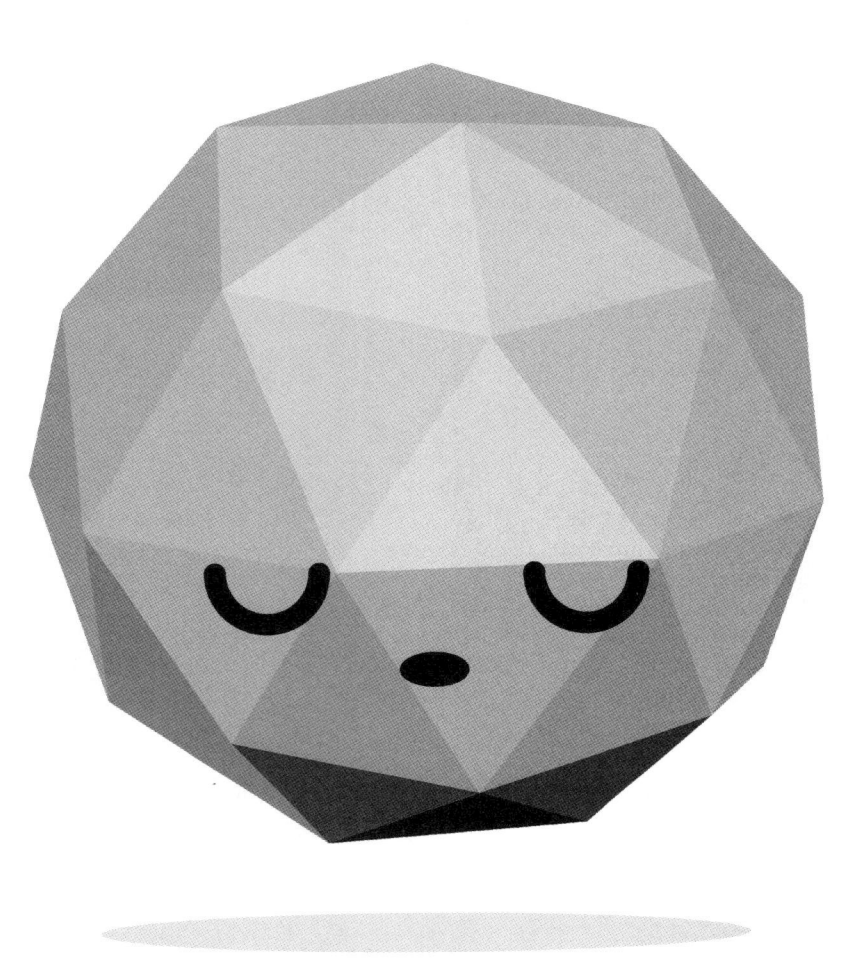

Chapter 5:
DEPRESSED, STRESSED, & ALL THE REST

> *If you just don't want to get out of bed, or feel as if life's burdens are coming at you all at once, I see you, and I'm here for you. The path forward may feel challenging, but there's a light at the end of the tunnel, and I can tell you, it's worth it!*

Whenever I am out and about, you will probably see me wearing some sort of The Drugless Doctors apparel. With this attire comes plenty of inquisitive stares, which often leads to many #AskDrBob questions. Can you guess what two of the top are? "Can you help me with mental distress and my anxiety?" and "What can I do for depression?"

Recently, I was contacted by a long-distance client who has been in and out of my life for quite a number of years. For this conversation, they just wanted to know if what they were currently doing was "right." This time, I could sense the desperation in her voice as she said, "Dr. Bob, I just finished suffering from a month of experiencing shingles. I don't feel the same. I have anxiety, my memory comes and goes, and I want to go back to how it used to be." My current default response, after the pleasantries of course, was to suggest an Omega Oils Serum Profile to determine her omega fat levels, in order to see how the brain fat is doing. (See Chapter Three).

During our initial consultation with patients, we explore every facet of health and their life with precision. This includes using a variety of tools, like various serum laboratory testing and written assessments, to discover what the most predominant challenge is: **depression**, anxiety, or both. Just the fact that we are listening and watching for subtle changes, we notice a difference in the whole appearance of someone with anxiety and depression compared to whatever we consider to be an "average" person.

With the addition of numerous technological devices today, researchers are creating an objective set of markers such as vocal tones, annunciations, facial expressions, and other behaviors. These devices use these markers much like we use vital signs to create a duplicable platform of one's mental state.

For example, right now a "red flag" for a mental or behavioral condition includes the fact that depressed patients have shorter smiles and move their heads less often. They look down more and don't enunciate vowels as much as those who do not have body signals of depression.

These are some of the indicators researchers have established using facial and acoustic analysis. With technology, they can measure shifts not always discernible to the eye or ear, such as slight movements of facial muscles as well as subtle changes in tone and language.

In my practice, I look at bodies to evaluate people's posture. While I am observing, I notice skin tone, sweat, hair integrity, skin tags, nail and lip chewing, bowed legs, and yes, body odor. There are countless lists of potential body markers that reveal so much about one's state of health.

Have you ever experienced a moment at a friend's or family member's house where there was a feeling of "tenseness" you could almost touch? After decades of practice, I am very aware after meeting a new patient for the first time, there is something which may be "off." It could be the word a person with anxiety might say, or someone who might be depressed, they won't even respond. (With this awareness, I want you to be thoughtful with what comes out of your mouth, in order to maintain the peace in your household, with coworkers, or with friends.)

> I would say that a good portion of individuals who have depression also experience anxiety.

Taking what I have experienced in my practice and one-on-one conversations, I would say that a good portion of individuals who have depression also experience anxiety. Not always, but more so than not. It is helpful to decide which condition is the principal one, since we administer protocols for each, but at the same time, we support the entire body. I have a two column self-evaluation of body signals for you to look at later in this chapter, which is one of the tools I use to get a sense of what is the predominant emotional status that is parallel to the supplement protocol need. (At our practice, we always follow the actual testing result numbers.)

Over the years, I have read statistics where up to 18% of the population has some sort of depression or anxiety concern, while in actuality, most people don't always realize when they are depressed or anxious. I care for a variety of patients who are raising grandchildren. I can see in their eyes a sense of despair because there seems to be no end in sight; they are exhausted and in a state of depression. I also have patients with chronic health challenges whether it be ear ringing, hands trembling, heart palpitations, or relentless pain for no apparent reason. They are absorbed with the pressures of life and have anxiety or a combination of both anxiety and depression.

Many individuals with depression may experience anxiousness or anxious distress because they have a continual sense of pressure and a heavy-burden feeling. This can take on the impression of constant trembling or even being fearful in every circumstance, in addition to their low mood. People with acute pain often feel tense, restless, and have trouble concentrating because of how much they actually worry, especially about their health.

These same individuals are extremely afraid something terrible is going to happen or they themselves might lose control. Individuals who experience this distress and depression may be at a higher risk for suicide, or need more intensive treatment. Sadly, it has been proposed about 10% of those with major depression symptoms take their own life, so it is essential to identify these anxious and disheartened body signals.

Anxiety and depression can occur literally at any age. Just because someone may look calm and healthy on the outside, does not mean they are quiet and stable on the inside. Pay attention to subtleties, especially one's voice. I am often surprised when I read or listen to testimonies and reviews about the experience someone who has visited our clinics has lived through. Many are eager to say they have less anxiety from when they first started under our care. Our patients often come in with a focus on chronic pain, not realizing this pain has created a fog around their perception of

> Just because someone may look calm and healthy on the outside, does not mean they are quiet and stable on the inside.

reality. Once we help diminish their pain, they realize they also had anxiety and may have been depressed. These feelings have finally lifted.

I recently had a gentleman who had poor focus capabilities and the ability to concentrate plagued him for a year—he works as a computer analyst. After his first visit to our office, he said the spinal correction to his upper cervical spine cleared his head and he was able to think clearly again. He did not even mention the lack of clarity on our first visit. Our evaluation included a motion radiographic study where we discovered locking and poor spinal function impaired brain to tissue cell communication.

Of recent observation, and of critical importance, is more teens and pre-teens with anxiety. Their comments to me often include conversation about their low-self-esteem and/or anger toward their parents who are not always part of their lives, because of life circumstances. Through these conversations, I also notice a competitive pressure causing anxiety in all age groups. In my practice, and around the US, there are more working women, this fact can create a hidden tension in their spouse's psyche. Many women today make more in their salary, which can be an ego-deflator for some men. This is only one indicator of many examples that result in distress.

In my own life, there was a situation where I did not catch someone's calls for help. There was a technologically advanced individual who was helping me with our computer systems at our practice and personal home devices. As he and I started to learn from one another, I discovered that he came from a family with a history of divorce, drugs, and alcohol. When he arrived for work at our practice on a Friday he said (and I can remember like it was yesterday), *"Dr. Bob, I need to talk to you."*

My response was, "I would love to, but I can't right now. I am seeing patients, and then will be on my way to the airport to catch a flight. Can we talk on Monday?"

> Make sure to watch for any changes in a person's countenance, stopping everything to save a life.

Well, Monday never came for him. That Friday night, he went over to his friend's house, parked his car outside, pulled the trigger, and shot himself. I have gone back over that scenario many times since. I didn't see the signals—and in today's world, we need to all pay attention a bit more. I am saying this now, so we all make sure to watch for any changes in a person's countenance, stopping everything to save a life.

Nowadays, this same type of scenario is becoming all-too familiar at our practice. I have parents who come into the office concerned their child is going to commit suicide and/or die of a recreational drug overdose, as they wring their hands in worry while talking about it. Technological advancements and devices have created another issue for our youth today: the amount of screen time someone has playing video games. The engineers who create these games have figured out the secret formula to make sure gamers come back for more and more. The video-game engineers have learned to stimulate the "addiction" centers of the players' brains so they want more. For example, parents and grandparents have told me their children ask for monetary gift cards so they can purchase virtual (not real or tangible) accessories to enhance their games. The video game industry is a multibillion-dollar conglomerate. One recent comment from a parent was, "I can tell my child, who is playing with blocks to go to bed, and they obediently listen, but if I tell my child who is playing video games the same thing, it is a resounding 'NOT RIGHT NOW, DAD!'" Addictive behavior can lead to unfulfilled expectations, and in the long run, create anxiety, depression, or both.

> Addictive behavior can lead to unfulfilled expectations, and in the long run, create anxiety, depression, or both.

Individuals who are depressed often do not share openly about their true inner feelings.

Yin and Yang

On another point, I am frequently asked by new and established patients about medical marijuana and **CBD oil** as part of a protocol for mental health and/or emotional issues, especially anxiety. They want to know if it can help. Personally, I prefer to begin with a lifestyle modification or "inside out" approach before recommending any non-food "outside in" modalities to achieve wellness.

In Traditional Chinese medicine (TCM), there are several philosophies regarding health and metabolism (see Chapter Four). There is a correlation between organs and your emotions. Chinese medicine has been around for thousands of years. When applied with a skilled practitioner, it can be beneficial, especially if the patient makes the necessary lifestyle changes to promote an environment of healing.

You may be hesitant about TCM, but its underlying principles, including yin and yang, play a significant role in emotional and physical health. I often refer to their guidelines when creating protocols for supplementation recommendations. We frequently use the principles and correlation of mental-emotional issues when helping to differentiate what the appropriate protocol may be since each person's condition and situation potentially requires a different remedy.

"All things exist as inseparable and contradictory opposites."

Yin and yang, in the realm of TCM, is that "all things exist as inseparable and contradictory opposites." Take for example female-male, dark-light, old-young. This TCM principle which dates from the third century BC, perhaps even earlier, is a fundamental concept in Chinese philosophy and culture. These two principles, with one being negative, dark, and feminine (yin), and one positive, bright, and masculine (yang), influence the life we live in nature.

Years ago, a scientist by the name of Dr. Royal Lee identified that members of the vitamin B complex had different, almost opposing properties. You can think of the features of the B vitamins as yin/yang. Dr. Lee broke them into a B fraction and a G fraction. The B fraction is more yang; vitamin B is primarily thiamin (B1) and pantothenic acid (B5), but also contains B4 and B12. The B faction causes **vasoconstriction** (small blood vessel diameter), increases muscle tone, improves low blood pressure, supports carbohydrate metabolism, and helps create hydrochloride for digestion.

Also, vitamin B aids the continuation and restoration of the sympathetic portion of your nervous system—the part of your nerves which speed you up when stressed and actually keeps your skin dry. There can be a combination of different levels of the B and G groups which is why some people can be depressed and have anxiety at the same time. Sugar depletes your body of vitamins and minerals, so you can understand how consuming it can sabotage even the best of intentions.

In contrast, vitamin G, the yin part of the B complex, supports the parasympathetic nervous system which slows the body down and when the dominant system, results in someone with excessive perspiration and more saliva in their mouth. The G part of the B complex is primarily riboflavin (B2) and niacin (B3), but PABA, folate, choline, inositol, and betaine are in this category as well. Vitamin G has an antispasmodic, tranquilizing, calming effect.

I have noticed those with adrenal gland fatigue and exhaustion and a dominant parasympathetic nervous system tend to have a subtle film of sweat on their skin and/or sweat profusely. Side note: I believe adrenal fatigue has fueled the antiperspirant industry.

Thiamin or B1 (yang) tends to be deficient in those who have feelings of impending doom, those patients who are anxious or have anxiety. Thiamin and other B vitamins are also depleted in individuals who consistently eat processed food. Vitamin B1 is also "destroyed" by some medications (antacids, birth control, and diuretics). People who are thiamin deficient tend to fall asleep for a short time and wake up, unable to go back to sleep. They are also prone and obsessed with negative thoughts, which is a significant point. They continuously use negative words when speaking about their future; I can perceive what is in their heart by listening to them for a short period of time. These are the people who consistently state the obvious to hear themselves: "I always catch a cold;" "I never have enough money;" "My car is junk." You get the idea, and hopefully, this is not you!

> Thiamin or B1 (yang) tends to be deficient in those who have feelings of impending doom, those patients who are anxious or have anxiety.

Assessing Vitamin B Needs

Now that you understand how specific nutrient deficiencies impact one's health, you can recognize why this is where I focus my attention when evaluating patients. If they, for example, are someone who goes to bed at 10 pm, I ask them if they wake up at any particular time regularly? The patient with a vitamin B1 deficiency may wake up one hour after going to sleep and then have a hard time going back to sleep. Those that wake at 3 am tend to have low blood sugar stress. If this is a female, she may experience hot flashes at the same time she is up. The question now is: did the hot flash wake her or was it the low blood sugar? Most of the time, it is the low blood sugar. Those waking up at 1 am may be agitated and get up because they have dysbiosis (gut flora) and parasites, which are active during this time of night. We initiate a vitamin B and blood sugar protocol product to assist those who wake up one hour or so after going to sleep.

Also, we can indirectly assess if someone needs vitamin B1 because they experience other body signals, including crying easily, mosquitoes are "attracted" to them, sore muscles after exercise, and positional dizziness.

Their mental body signals specifically would include: apprehensiveness, being detached from reality, and intolerance to noise. I have noticed a lot of females have noise sensitivity with "raw nerves," which is having pain in various tissues. They can hear the humming of a refrigerator from a distant room while their partner does not understand or recognize any such noise.

On a serum blood test, we notice the carbon dioxide (CO_2) may be characteristically low in the proximity range of twenty when looking at the scale, which can be eighteen to thirty depending on the lab reference scale used. This may suggest, and based on other factors like gasping for air and itchy skin, the body is in a state of acid or low pH with a need for vitamin B1. Patients who have low blood pressure or blood pressure that drops from a sit to stand position may thrive with vitamin B1. I also have noticed when using the Heart Sound Recorder (an electronic stethoscope placed over the heart valves on the chest), there is a wider gap in the heart sounds of someone who does not have enough vitamin B1. So, you can see how someone with anxiety can also have chest pain and/or heart symptoms, including a speeding heart or tachycardia.

The other part of the vitamin B spectrum (the yin) includes choline and riboflavin. The mental correlations with the yin deficiency includes excessive worry, apprehension, moodiness, depression, and raised suspicion.

Choline is a fat emulsifier that assists the liver in processing fat and is a precursor of acetylcholine for the brain. We recommend phosphatidyl-choline to our patients who have emotional distress in the late summer and early fall with the labeled condition: Seasonal Affective Disorder (SAD). This product has been very useful and a favorable option in lieu of an anti-depressant. Phosphatidylcholine is excellent for nerve function, and you will notice the choline portion is outstanding for optimal fat metabolism necessary for healthy brain and nervous system functionality. It is a source for a brain neurotransmitter called acetylcholine.

I may also suggest phosphatidylcholine to my patients who have Alzheimer's, Parkinson's, senility, neuromuscular disorders (multiple sclerosis, myositis, nerve pain), synaptic dysfunction (seen in memory loss), elevated blood fats, fatty liver, gallbladder symptoms, gallstones, migraine headaches, and adrenal fatigue. You can see this is a pretty remarkable product. When our patients are under extreme mental stress, we often encourage them to consider taking a trace mineral called lithium. The product we use is sourced from plants and is metabolized in the gut to produce acetylcholine which is required for optimal brain function. The puzzle for optimal mental health includes an often overlooked optimal functioning gut.

Recently at our practice, a grandmother called Mary (not her real name) was referred by her friend Rita. Rita came to visit us first with a feeling of anxiousness but decided to go all in and change her diet, begin exercising, and also receive spinal nervous system remedial care. Within one month, years of anxiety and chest pain along with a deep breathing condition disappeared!

Rita was so excited that she encouraged Mary to visit us. When we started Mary's care, she had a forward posture, which reduces the oxygen available by restricting the diaphragm impairing brain function. After our initial consultation, she asked if I was going to "cure" her. She had high expectations because her friend had a new sense of happiness. I told Mary I did not cure anyone, but I would be her guide on her journey. Mary went on to say along with her depression and stomach pain, her daughter was getting divorced, which added to her stress level. Well, Mary did respond— she stopped her sugar consumption, and we added the correct high potency yang portion of the B vitamins.

She was doing so good, then she cut back on her B vitamins herself and went back to indulging in sugar; so much so, her relationship with her daughter became bitter and combative. Her pattern is not unusual as many others who are on their journey have unpredictable highs and lows. Changing your own supplementation and going back to crippling habits will deny you of the victory you seek. Stay on the path, and always consult your health care practitioner of changes you desire to make.

Please listen here: we all have stress. If I would share with you the stress that I deal with daily, you might need a vacation. Hear me out, from the bottom of my heart, stop consuming sugar. Instead, focus on whatever protocol or combination is required to sustain your health.

Self-Evaluation Assessment

Now, I have a self-evaluation assessment for you to look at, which will help narrow down what part of the B vitamin family your body may need. It can be weighted more on one side than the other. Look at all the body signals: this will help create a protocol for anxiety or a combination of depression and anxiety.

DIFFERENCES BETWEEN "B" & "G"

B/Yang
Please check all that apply:

General Correlations:
- ❏ Frequently bitten by mosquitoes
- ❏ Decreased body temperature
- ❏ Low blood pressure
- ❏ Need muscle tone
- ❏ Improper carbohydrate metabolism
- ❏ Small blood vessels
- ❏ Inhibition of thyroid (many low hypothyroid symptoms)

Heart Correlations:
- ❏ Slow heartbeat or pulse
- ❏ Irregular heartbeat

Digestive Correlations:
- ❏ Acid pH
- ❏ Irregular salivary glands
- ❏ Lack of appetite
- ❏ Drowsiness after meals

Mental Correlations:
- ❏ Increased psychotic tendencies
- ❏ Apprehensiveness
- ❏ Intolerance to noise

Neurological Correlations:
- ❏ Lack of vibration sense
- ❏ Headaches like a tight band around head
- ❏ Burning in soles of feet
- ❏ Tenderness in calves

Sleep Difficulty Correlations:
- ❏ Frequent nighttime urination
- ❏ Awakens and cannot return to sleep
- ❏ Back pain – especially at night

Female Estrogen Metabolism:
- ❏ Spider nevi – veins on legs
- ❏ Breast swelling with menses
- ❏ Premenstrual water retention
- ❏ Long, heavy period
- ❏ Short intervals between periods
- ❏ Generalized bloating

Respiratory Correlations:
- ❏ Decreased breath holding time
- ❏ Shortness of breath
- ❏ Decreased respiratory rate

Adrenal Correlations:
- ❏ Bright light bothers eyes
- ❏ Sluggish or frequently tired
- ❏ Frequent yawning
- ❏ Dizziness from sit to stand position

G/Yin
Please check all that apply:

General Correlations:
- ❏ Menstrual cramps
- ❏ Muscle cramps
- ❏ High blood pressure
- ❏ Up-tight / high-strung
- ❏ Improper fat metabolism
- ❏ Large blood vessels

Heart Correlations:
- ❏ Heart races – Tachycardia
- ❏ Chest Pain – Pre-angina pectoris

Digestive Correlations:
- ❏ Alkaline pH
- ❏ Digestive distress
- ❏ Spastic gallbladder – cucumbers, onion & peppers cause distress
- ❏ Pass gas

Mental Correlations:
- ❏ Excessively worried
- ❏ Apprehensive
- ❏ Moody
- ❏ Depressed
- ❏ Suspicious

Neurological Correlations:
- ❏ Restless legs – jumpy, shaky legs
- ❏ Seasonal Affective Disorder (SAD)

Sleep Difficulty Correlations:
- ❏ Whole body or limb jerks
- ❏ Can hear heartbeat on pillow

Skin & Mucous Membrane Correlations:
- ❏ Cracking at corners of mouth (cheilosis)
- ❏ Irritated skin – especially on face and neck (after shaving)
- ❏ Bright red tip of tongue
- ❏ Strawberry tongue (purple)
- ❏ Thin upper lip
- ❏ Irritated mucous membranes: rectum, vagina, eyes (frequent watering)

Visual Correlations:
- ❏ Burning or itching of eyes
- ❏ Light bothers eyes
- ❏ Eyelid spasm
- ❏ Bloodshot eyes
- ❏ See only parts of printed words
- ❏ When viewing, items have a fishbowl effect

With the insight you have gathered from the personal nutritional body signal evaluation, you can now check your current mental status. Traditionally in the office, those who have a predominant amount of checks on the left column tend to have anxiety; those on the right column potentially can be more depressed. What is essential is that you can have a combination of the two, and this is why we see patients with characteristics of both. With proper supplementation and personal food choice selection, the body signals can improve.

> With proper supplementation and personal food choice selection, the body signals can improve.

Physical body signals of depression:

- **Unhappy disposition**
- **Lack of interest in enjoyable activities**
- **Increase or decrease in appetite**
- **Insomnia or hypersomnia (can sleep anytime)**
- **Slowing of movement (no "jump" in one's step)**
- **Lack of energy (one of the most common body signals of depressed people)**
- **Feelings of guilt or insignificance**
- **Trouble concentrating**
- **Suicidal thoughts or behaviors**

For a diagnosis of major depressive disorder from what I have studied and read, someone theoretically experiences five or more of these indicators for at least two weeks. In my honest opinion, most people in this category have experienced these for months or years and they just do not know what to do about it or who to talk to.

The majority of female patients I have seen with emotional distress have suffered for a long time. Some individuals began their experience with the onset of their menses at an early age and thought it was normal. Others who have children start with postpartum depression, which is a common condition. Interestingly enough, as I was writing this book, there was a headline released saying there were new potential prescription medications for **postpartum depression**. (Of course it has to do with drugs!) The way it worked was unknown, and by the way, would cost between twenty and thirth-five thousand US dollars per year!

I am seeing more and more individuals who become depressed because they believe the smokescreen of others in their social media universe. They get trapped into thinking they will never achieve apparent expectations and/or they are looking for more validation when it comes to relationships. I bring this up because as humans, we are wired to be social. It is very interesting when I look at my social media "friends" with selfies, vacation locations, and pictures of painted toenails on lounge chairs and what they are trying to portray. I have seen celebrities who constantly post pictures of themselves looking for validation.

In the ever-evolving social world, both past and present, you might not be considered "healthy" if you don't have a life partner. As our culture is transitioning, there is a shift, with more individuals content with being single. I have also witnessed more single adults over the age of fifty, who are single because of a divorce or the passing of a spouse, develop depression. These factors are a setup for the high anxiety or depressed merry-go-round. The social media world and generational perception is changing the landscape on how life is perceived as happy or content. I am sure many feel a true personal connection with others on social media and even have connected by dating and developing lifelong relationships.

Did you score more on the left side of the assessment? It is possible you may have anxiety. I have a list of typical anxiety body signals.

Physical body signals of Anxiety:

- **Excessive worry (most common)**
- **Restlessness or impatience**
- **Easily fatigued**
- **Having trouble concentrating**
- **Irritability**
- **Sleep disturbances**
- **Muscle tension**
- **May have chest and neck pain (grabbing one's chest, especially on the left side)**

If you have experienced these symptoms on most days for more than six months, and the other body signals I discussed in the yang B vitamin list are creating distress in your daily life, then you may receive a diagnosis of generalized anxiety disorder. Other types of anxiety disorders include separation anxiety, panic disorder, and phobias. I have noticed both with adults and children that separation anxiety is a real, physical challenge today because of divorce. This can be actual or perceived parental abandonment with biological parents who focused on themselves versus raising and training their children.

The actual phobias and panic disorders can be managed and resolved with the right nutritional supplementation, which I recommend after evaluating the entire picture, including whole-body lifestyle patterns. It is significant to look at the whole picture: relationships, family history, work history, addictive patterns, stress levels, and current geographical location. Some people are not joyful in the cold north while others are not cheerful in the sunny, warm south. Thyroid function does impact a person's response to the effects of hot and cold weather on the body. I also use the results from serum blood tests, saliva, and urine metabolite evaluation.

For example, hormonal imbalances with an excessive increase or an imbalance of estrogen and progesterone in ladies, or low testosterone in men, can disrupt mental stability. Creating a lifestyle pattern for the body to work on its own without interference is the goal. You will not lose weight and keep it off if you continue to fill the cookie jar or purchase snacks you passionately desire to devour in your living quarters.

> Creating a lifestyle pattern for the body to work on its own without interference is the goal.

I also have historically noticed men in their late thirties and early forties (most common age demographic for men in our practice) who are on some sort of medication to "take the edge off." This age demographic is where I find men struggling to mentally cope with their personal health, work, and family responsibilities.

The most common age group for women at our practice is between ages thirty-seven and forty-three with two kids. This is because their bodies have changed hormonally after carrying two children and the impact it has on their physical being along with the emotional toll of raising their children while balancing marriage, parents, and work.

If you compare the two lists of symptoms mentioned above, you can see that there is some overlap. Sleep problems, trouble concentrating, and fatigue are all symptoms of both anxiety and depression. Irritability may also manifest in forms of anxiety or depression, in place of a "low" mood.

Recently, I had an opportunity to help three young ladies, two of whom were sisters. All three had anxiety and stress. One of the three, I determined had a blood sugar issue. According to her mom, she was always hungry but does not take the time to prepare food to have available while traveling (they drove an hour each way to our practice). At the time of my conversation with her, she did have a blood sugar challenge and had her mom stop and purchase something for her to eat. She chose ranch-flavored corn chips.

I politely showed her and the sibling what each of the ingredients in those chips meant. In this case, the oils listed were: sunflower and canola. Having the correct oils in your body (see Chapter Three) impacts nervous system function and can sabotage mental alertness. I did discuss with the family that part of their challenge was the food they were eating, or not eating. So, in other words, when I read their diet sheet, it was loaded with grains, sugar, poor oil choices, and dairy. These choices created an imbalance with excessive omega-6 oils. We did complete an Omega Oils Serum Profile test on her, and she was low in the brain-friendly and healthy long-chain fat, DHA.

This family, like so many, is addicted to food groups that compromise brain health. We have been assessing omega fats for years. I can confidently say, most of the patients I see, who think they are making the correct choices, actually have an imbalance: too much omega-6 compared to omega-3 fats with increased inflammatory linoleic and arachidonic fats. (Go to page 9, Chart #1 to review the Omega-6 Fatty Acids.) People are choosing too many foods labeled all-natural or organic which have excessive inflammatory oils such as sunflower and safflower oils

Irritability can also be caused by a relatively new state of distress called "hangry." There are those individuals who have low blood sugar emotional distress, including anger. Over the years, I have witnessed mental suffering with occurrences of low blood sugar (formally and currently labeled hypoglycemia) which is relieved with, of course, sugar. For whatever reason, hypoglycemia emotional distress is not commonly discussed. When your blood sugar drops after either ingesting too much sugar with an insulin spike or not eating, your brain is looking for energy without which you may start to experience anger, brain fog, confusion, and mental distress.

Lifestyle Features

As we progress in our study of depression and anxiety, there are some distinguishing lifestyle features between the two. Those with depression move more slowly, and their reactions can seem flattened or dulled. I have seen friends and acquaintances who move slow and deliberate. I know of a gentleman in his mid-seventies who is directing a business he inherited through marriage. His father-in-law passed on, so he assumed the responsibility of continuing the business. Well, now he wants to sell the company, but unbeknownst to him, at first, his sister-in-law is on the payroll. She does not work, yet expects to be financially compensated because she feels entitled, since it was a family business. (You could probably fit your story in here also.)

This fine gentleman is so out of sorts and depressed, he does not know what to do. He always has something going on with his health, and he does not have an "out"—he is slow and exhausted. I suggested to his wife they have a meeting to sort this out, or he could break under the pressure and experience a complete meltdown. There are so many people like him who do not confront what is interrupting their life. There is no spring to their step and no energy in their countenance.

People with anxiety tend to be more keyed up as they struggle to manage their racing thoughts. I have many anxious patients who look like they're going to snap. Mom's with high energy, who are doing their best to create the perfect life for their family, are exhausted from working which, in turn, leads to no libido, medication, and surgical interventions, such as breast augmentation for cosmetic purposes. They are searching for happiness through all of these outside factors—but what is going on inside?

Those experiencing anxiety tend to always have a fear about the future, whereas those with depression are less likely to be fearful of future events, since they do not experience apprehension. People with anxiety are often resigned to believing things will continue to be wrong. In their words, they may predict the future based on how they feel at the moment. I often think of Charlie Brown and Eeyore as the poster characters for this example.

> Those experiencing anxiety tend to always have a fear about the future, whereas those with depression are less likely to be fearful of future events, since they do not experience apprehension.

I have also witnessed more and more, during the last almost twenty years, grandparents raising their grandchildren. Some of this is by the abandonment of biological parents because of drug addiction, death by overdose, or an inability to handle raising their children. I have seen many families at my practice experience the dynamics of their family structure interrupted due to a death by suicide.

There is also a direct link to depression in those individuals who have altered fat metabolism, which we have talked about in the chapter about supporting brain health. When DHA is low, from either not supplementing or choosing the wrong food choice, depression can occur. Ladies tend to have postpartum depression because their liver-gallbladder loop has been altered. The gallbladder and liver work together to make sure fat is ready to be delivered to all body units, including the brain and nervous system. When you have digestive distress and bloating two or three hours after eating, and/or digestive distress with onions, garlic, radishes, and cucumbers, it is possible your liver-gallbladder mechanism is not processing oils properly. You can have mental distress because of this backlog. I would make sure you are eating at least one half of a red apple daily, which helps promote adequate bile flow. I also talked about the liver and gallbladder in the emotional correlation of glandular function. (Please see Chapter Three to read about the thyroid, tyrosine, and mental health and depression.)

Creating Healthy Dialogue

I'd like to conclude this chapter with how to create a healthy dialogue with a friend or family member who has depression or anxiety in order to "be there" for them.

Depression is real and there are a number of individuals who are depressed. I personally have never been depressed, so I do not know what a depressed person "feels" like, but I see it every day in my practice. My wife told me she was depressed back when she was in high school and early on in our marriage during times of transition. We worked together with diet changes, exercise, minimizing alcohol, and instruction into and growing in our faith walk.

With observation, at my clinic and outside of it, you cannot flippantly say to someone in this condition, "You will be OK" or "Just snap out of it." You must take time with them. If you say you are going to check up on them—DO IT. I believe with all sincerity, there are dietary and possibly relationship reasons for depression. I know, because of my experience, having the right oil and cofactors is critically essential for proper mental/brain health. Taking an antidepressant is not going to cure you, it may manage symptoms, but "curing" is going to require establishing the proper physiology.

One of the biggest challenges I contend with are those who read my other books and tell me there is no cure for ADHD, depression, or anxiety. This saddens me because I know for a fact it is not true. It's like they are carrying it as a "crutch." I just had someone who has been in my life for over forty years tell me that her husband did not want to change his situation. He takes nine different medications a day; he is depressed and even had Botox injections for headaches. She looked me square in the eye and said, "I believe my husband is using his health challenge as an excuse." She then smiled and walked away. Point made!

*This chapter is dedicated to
the memory of Mike.*

Helpful Reminders

- Review the characteristics of depression and anxiety. Are you focused on one area more than the other, or both?

- Consider having an Omega Oils Serum Profile to evaluate your oil levels to see if your long-chain brain fat DHA level is within normal range.

- Consider the Organix™ Urine Test to assess your carbohydrate, fat and protein metabolism metabolites. Also your potential L-Tyrosine and other toxic and deficiency chemicals and nutrients are evaluated with the Organix™ Test.

- Request a Thyroid Panel with TSH, T3, T4, and TPO to evaluate thyroid function.

- Eat a variety of organic plant and animal protein. Avoid eating sugar and soy products.

- Avoid omega-6 fats (safflower and sunflower) and read labels. Use olive oil for your salad dressing.

- Reduce stress and consider an adrenal adaptogen for stress management.

- Do not overcommit your time, which increases your stress level.

- If you have a friend who is depressed, stick with them. If you are depressed, share this book with someone so they can understand what your life is like.

- Look for an accountability partner to walk your life path with. Learn to trust and become vulnerable with someone—you may find it benefits you both!

- Take the B (Yang) G (Yin) Assessment and supplement accordingly.

Chapter Glossary

All definitions were sourced from the *Merriam-Webster Dictionary* unless otherwise noted.

CBD—A nonintoxicating cannabinoid found in cannabis and hemp

Depression—A mood disorder marked especially by sadness, inactivity, difficulty in thinking and concentration, a significant increase or decrease in appetite and time spent sleeping, feelings of dejection and hopelessness, and sometimes suicidal tendencies; a state of feeling sad

Seasonal Affective Disorder—Depression that tends to recur chiefly during the late fall and winter and is associated with shorter hours of daylight

Tachycardia—Relatively rapid heart action whether physiological (as after exercise) or pathological

Vasoconstriction—Narrowing of the lumen of blood vessels

Patient Testimonial

"Years ago, I was just going through life's motions. To help with depression, I was put on Prozac and Zoloft, and took each for several years. To an extent, they may have changed my behavior, but did not get to the root of the issue. I was feeling the effects of the medication, as I was more lethargic and not living each day to its fullness. That is when I came to visit Dr. DeMaria and through his suggested blood testing, found out that my thyroid was low. I followed his supplementation plan, and have now been off medication for ten years! I have more energy, vitality, and mental clarity. Life couldn't be any better!"

– M.S.

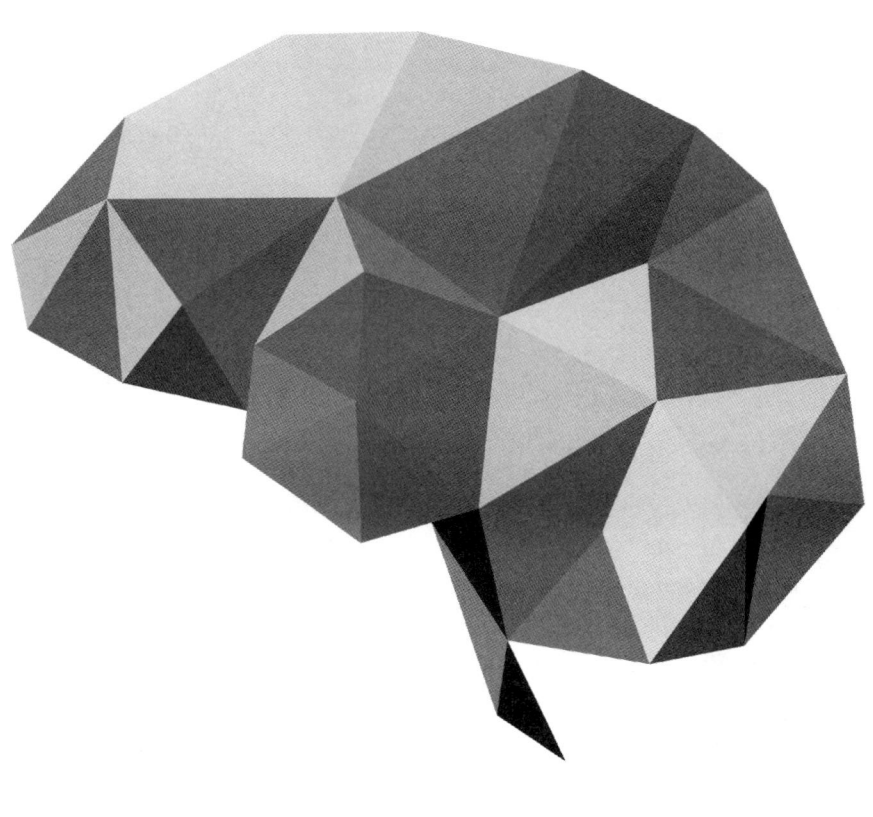

Chapter 6:
LET'S TAKE A WALK DOWN MEMORY LANE

Imagine for a moment: you're attending a well-known conference and anticipating the keynote presentation to begin. The speaker challenges, motivates, and brings encouragement. As everyone is leaving, there across the room is someone who seems to notice you as they walk towards you with a broad smile. With their arms open wide, you're at a loss. "Who are you?" Even still, they embrace you as if you were a member of their family. As you are mentally going through your database of everyone you may have ever encountered, nothing registers.

Sometimes, our memory lapses are as simple as recalling a single word. Other times, you don't even remember a close friend or family member. Any experience with memory recollection causes concern, embarrassment, and even anxiety. If you relate to any of these, this chapter is for you!

Our body, brain, and neurological systems, all "socialize" together, interacting with a variety of communication messages all working collectively in unison. There is also a variety of interdependent chemical, hormonal, and neurologic systems along with networks in your body, whose primary goal is to create optimal messaging and cellular function. Nerves are the vehicles in which actual electrical signals or messages are sent from the brain to the rest of your body, instructing every interchange and decision you need to make in order to live a quality life.

Like I mentioned above, our bodies work together in unity for the good of the whole. Nerve tissue, as with all the other components of the communication network, are dependent on wise food choices and manageable stress practices to operate at full capacity. The objective is to keep the connections between the nerves, or synapses, unbroken without "clutter" or missteps.

> Our bodies work together in unity for the good of the whole.

Our bodies have named nervous systems; one is the **central nervous system**, or CNS. The CNS consists of your brain and spinal cord. The outer portion of the brain or cortex portion is protected by the skull (cranial cavity). The spinal cord travels from the lower part of the brain protected by the mobile spinal column. This is the central portion ending in the lumbar region of the lower back and continuing on to all nerve fibers.

Another system which is not discussed often is in your gut, named the **enteric nervous system** (ENS). The ENS is an independent part of the nervous system and includes nerve routes controlling motor function, local blood flow, mucosal transport (linings of the intestine), and secretions. It controls the immune and endocrine functions. It's also known as a "second brain," since it has its own reflexes and is independent of the brain and spinal cord. The ENS impacts digestion and, in a roundabout way, is a critical player in mental health.

I want you to think about this: if you have digestive distress (commonly called acid indigestion) and go to a traditional physician, you will more than likely be prescribed a drug to neutralize the acid interrupting stomach health, often without any tests. The drug you are now going to be taking for a long time will potentially cause mental health issues and/or memory problems in the future. Your body will not absorb the necessary nutrients, cofactors, fats, minerals, and B vitamins if you do not have proper digestion.

A good portion of the activity in your body, keeping you alive and functioning at 100%, occurs automatically via a group of nerves named the **autonomic nervous system** (ANS). The ANS is composed of two portions; one of these systems is called the **sympathetic nervous system** (SNS). This system can sometimes speed the body up by placing a demand on the adrenal glands. Your adrenals are located on top of the kidneys and help manage hormone production when you are stressed by releasing glucocorticoids, stress-related hormones. The counterpart to the sympathetic function is the **parasympathetic nervous system** (PNS). The PNS regulates the production of gastric acid in the stomach, which impacts overall digestive health. Can you begin to see the connection?

The sympathetic nervous system is continuously called on to execute whenever we find ourselves in a stressful situation. This system is on continuous alert as we live out our "always on" life.

> The sympathetic nervous system is continuously called on to execute whenever we find ourselves in a stressful situation.

The SNS also has a consistent demand placed on it to speed up the whole body. This speeding up is attributed to actual or perceived stress. This overtaxing pattern can wear your body down. Adrenal exhaustion is a common result of ongoing SNS activity. This scenario can then be sabotaged by a mineral deficiency. For example, a zinc deficiency is commonly associated with memory loss. The deficiency can occur in part from an abundant amount of wheat consumption (daily and sometimes with each meal), soy, which interrupts absorption, or sugar. Consuming these cannibalizes nearly all the body's minerals as it attempts to balance its own pH. This cycle can deteriorate into a state of inflammation, as if your body is a building on fire. A deficiency in zinc impacts the portion of your brain that manages short and long-term memory called the hippocampus. With a zinc deficiency, you have the potential to experience memory and mental lapses.

To achieve optimal function, your nerves require a continual source of a particular, preferred long-chain fatty acid oil called DHA (see Chapter One). I discovered in the 1980's a specific type of oil (trans fat or partially hydrogenated oil) had its original structural chemistry altered interrupting the normal flow of information along nerve fibers, much like an alteration in thin, glass fiber optic wires.

One of my degrees is in human biology. When I was in postgraduate school, I wanted to improve my hands-on experience on how the human body actually functions. With that in mind, I became a "gross" anatomy lab instructor, meaning I trained students in human dissection. Earlier on, as one of the anatomy students, I was tested by my lab instructors using a straight pin labeled with a number attached to it and placed in strategic anatomy parts. For example, on a nerve fiber in a cadaver, I was required to name the nerve or anatomical structure the pin was placed on or in.

As life would have it, I recently had the misfortune of a fiber optic cable breaking at the outer shell of the modem in our house. This meant instantly, there was absolutely no communication with the outside world via this cable. Our technician-to-the-rescue shared that this cable carries massive amounts of information at high speeds. The optic "wire" was actually smaller than the named nerves from my anatomy lab. Interestingly enough, I could not even fathom placing a straight pin in the fiber optic glass, that's how small it was. This is the counterpart to the nerves inside our body. So, imagine what happens during the breakdown in your own communication headquarters.

I believe most people think nerves in their own bodies are microscopic, but in reality, they are quite large. The sciatic nerve, for example, is located in your low back, which travels into the buttocks and legs; it can be the size of your thumb! Nerves carry important information while neurochemical transmitters carry information throughout the entire human body. Every single cell is connected via either a chemical or nerve wiring.

Fear of Memory Loss

When I'm listening to my patients, one of the biggest "real-life" fears is losing their ability to remember. Just yesterday, as I was writing this, someone shared with me they were concerned they would "get" Alzheimer's or **dementia** like their parents before them. This thought brings more new would-be patients into our practice than those who only casually desire to get healthy. The health and healing mindset today is based on the fear of the unknown, and doing what they can so as not to become like their "memory-compromised" parents.

> The health and healing mindset today is based on the fear of the unknown.

This was actually the case with my own mother, who succumbed to memory loss. She passed without the ability to identify scrambled eggs on her plate, nor did she realize you were to actually *eat* them. All of this to say, my mom had a life passion, and that passion's name was sugar. She loved sugar in all of its shapes and sizes. Growing up, we even had a large rooster cookie jar always filled with cookies, and right next to it was a metal-covered pan with some sort of frosted cake waiting to be devoured. My dad always made sure there was plenty of chocolate and sodas available also. They were both raised during the Great Depression of the 1930's and did not want their children to miss out on the "better" things in which they could not enjoy growing up.

As for my mother-in-law, she loved to eat fatty foods and always made a point to go out and grab a sandwich. Not only a sandwich, but one loaded with fatty deli meats, melted cheese, and topped with mayonnaise. She did not pass with memory loss. Unfortunately, she passed from a massive cardiovascular event precipitated by her food choices. Her memory was intact till the end, unlike my mom, who suffered from memory loss for years prior to passing.

The fact is, every day I witness the negative impact sugar causes to one's health by depleting essential mineral cofactors, such as zinc, in their **The food you eat becomes you.** bodies. You must realize the food you eat becomes you. When not chosen properly, the wrong food can interrupt normal physiology in your body. I personally have thought people know what they are supposed to eat to support their health. But because I have seen thousands of patient food journals, people may hear or read about good foods, but many choose to ignore what is optimal. In addition, reading labels can also be confusing, leading consumers to just "stick with what they know" regardless if it negatively impacts their health.

WHO Guidelines

Recently, the World Health Organization[1] released their first set of guidelines, after years of silence which could have prevented early brain dysfunction along with the disruption of entire families. These recommendations are designed to reduce the risk of dementia and cognitive decline, while highlighting dementia as a global health priority. The suggested recommendations seek to help people limit the risk of dementia and cognitive decline through interventions, such as increased physical activity, reduced alcohol, and weight management.

The guidelines went on to suggest that dementia and memory loss is not necessarily an inevitable part of aging. Quite the eye opener is the fact that there is now an estimated fifty million people around the world who are suffering from some sort of mental dysfunction with an additional ten million being added each year. By the year 2030, it will cost around two trillion dollars a year to manage the price of memory loss. The author of the article also went on to mention there is no known cure for dementia, with the typical suggestions being to eat a healthy diet, reduce alcohol consumption, manage blood sugar, and one's weight.

Through my observations, what they are suggesting is not a cure. If you look around, you too will notice over half of the population in the United States is twenty pounds or more overweight. It was estimated that at the turn of the millennium, 30% of those born in the year 2000 would have diabetes by 2030. The typical, healthy diet includes the word "moderation," which makes me chuckle. Who has discipline when there is the allowance of moderation? One of the leading causes of inflammation, including a fatty liver, is the amount of fruit and supposedly "healthy" dairy products included. The bottom line is: inflammation is the key to altered physiology, leading to a variety of health challenges, including memory impairment.

> Inflammation is the key to altered physiology, leading to a variety of health challenges, including memory impairment.

I'm sure you are aware there is always a new fad diet rising to popularity on social and traditional media, whereas in reality, people do not know what they should or should not be eating for optimal health. Recently, it has been celery juice, bone broths, Whole 30, intermittent fasting, Keto, and more. In reality, eating healthy and correctly is pretty simple. Focus on whole foods which are non-starchy and organic green vegetables that are prepared by being steamed, sautéed, baked, or eaten raw. It's important to always expand your food choices, so you're not eating the same thing every day. I do suggest, if your budget allows, purchasing organic meat. If you choose to be plant-based, do not get yourself hooked on eating excessive grains and starches without the right blend of amino acids or protein building blocks.

The combination of sugar consumption and stress interrupts significant cofactors, which are essential ingredients used to complete metabolic pathways. These include larger minerals, such as magnesium and zinc, and trace minerals, such as lithium and chromium, all of which are necessary ingredients required by the body to complete healthy fat and nervous system function. Stress interrupts cofactors because they tend to lower the pH in the body making it acidic. I want you to compare vinegar to what an acid is. When the body is in an acidic state, it does its best to raise the pH number (a measure of acidity and alkalinity). The opposite of acid is called alkaline, the body will take minerals and other nutrients from structures in the body, like bones, to neutralize its acid state.

This is why, for example, someone with stress tends to get cold sores. It's because stress depletes calcium and having enough available is very important for "gluing" cell membranes together. When you have a shortage of calcium, a virus can do its dirty work by penetrating between cell membranes, resulting in a painful, itchy lesion on your lip. I know this from experience, because I used to get them in the past until I learned to take my calcium and L-Lysine daily.

When it comes to memory loss, no one has come up with an exact metabolic reason we have a retention issue. Some scholars allude to the fact there may be plaque on the brain. Others say it is reduced blood flow. Others still think it is aluminum toxicity. I am sure there are others now who are reading this and have their own theories while continuing to search for answers.

I believe the critical challenge for most, if not all, of our mental health concerns, including memory impairment, is inflammation caused by an altered fat metabolism of DHA and the omega-3 fat metabolic pathway. This, along with a deficiency of essential nutrients, or cofactors, and a deficiency of vitamin B12 can lead to memory loss. DHA production can be interrupted from poor food choices. Eating processed foods sabotages the creation of DHA via a brain-fat metabolic pathway. Choosing to consume artificial or natural pro-inflammatory items, especially dairy and gluten, are creating deficiencies that increase the need for medications, which alter the absorption of critically-needed nutrients. Typically, it is a combination of all of these.

Consider this scenario: Former President Ronald Regan had Alzheimer's and dementia. He also had a passion for jellybeans. They even spent thousands of dollars at his inauguration to make sure there were plenty of jellybeans available for guests.

Right now, yes now, I would like *you* to evaluate the direction *you* are going. Are the choices you are making able to sustain you with optimal brain function? Or, will you end up in a facility like my mom, who if you can remember, did not know what the food on her plate was?

You may want to ask me, "Dr. Bob, are *you* not concerned you will have Alzheimer's like your mom?"

My answer is a resounding NO. Debbie and I decided when we first married in 1976 that we were not going to use our family's recipe boxes.

Instead, we opted for a plant-based diet with organic animal protein, no alcohol, and no sugar. I do use organic half and half in my organic coffee. Neither of us smokes, nor uses artificial sweeteners.

Alzheimer's, dementia, and/or memory loss does not care what social or economic layer you come from. There are rules, or physiological principles, one must adhere to. If you follow simple physiological guidelines, you will have a better chance to stay mentally stable to the end, with healthy mental acuity.

If you are continually placing a physiological demand on your nervous system by eating sugar, using an abundance of inflammatory omega-6 fats, making poor processed food choices, or overusing chemicals on your body (lotions, shampoos, etc.), you will have some sort of adverse collateral damage, which may include a cardiovascular incident or memory loss.

I would like to discuss several reasons for memory loss, and yes, there is more than one. There are actually a number of explanations. I do not want to claim I have all the answers, but I do know I have been practicing in "drugless healthcare" long before it was popular to be a natural or functional practitioner. Food does impact your function. I have listened to, studied, investigated, and more the hundreds of thousands of patients I've seen in my office. Here is a perspective of my experience in order for you to see why I am explaining what I have discovered.

There is a portion of your brain called the hippocampus, and it is essential for memory function, particularly the transfer from short to long-term memory. It is also one of the few areas of the brain capable of growing new nerve cells, called neurons.

What is interesting is the hippocampus requires zinc to function optimally. Without zinc, there will be an increase in the stress-related glucocorticoids.[2] This is part of the inflammation issue we all contend with throughout our day, and why individuals who are stressed may have the potential to have declining health, along with memory difficulties. Zinc is also necessary for the production of the long-chain fat, DHA, which is needed by the brain and nervous system for memory.

Zinc Deficiencies & Mental Health

As we continue our stroll down memory lane, let me share with you some real-life clinical truths about zinc.

It can be depleted by eating wheat and soy. Soy is often used as a protein filler disguised as texturized protein and has been touted for decades as a viable source of protein for those primarily choosing to be "plant" eaters. I have never promoted soy—just check out my "Shake My Head" videos on social media. For those of you who are only "plant-based," change the soy, including tofu, to broad-leafed kale and red quinoa for protein. In my observations, the general public loves to eat wheat-based everything (pizza, pasta, bread). Those who primarily consider themselves to be plant-eaters tend to have more copper in their body, which is antagonistic to zinc. A good source of zinc I have found is pumpkin seeds.

> Those who primarily consider themselves to be plant-eaters tend to have more copper in their body, which is antagonistic to zinc.

At our practice and from the beginning of my professional days, we have completed a Mineral Tissue Hair Analysis which lately makes me feel like I'm starring on *CSI*, since this analysis can be likened to forensic medicine. It uses new hair growth, from the nape of the neck to establish results. Your hair sample is evaluated by an analytical research laboratory. I typically notice elevated copper compared to zinc on the individuals suffering from a variety of health challenges, including blood sugar stress, enlarged prostates, large facial pores, loss or diminished sense of smell and taste, white spots on the nails, and neurologic challenges, including ADHD, depression, and memory loss.

We also complete a Zinc Taste Test with individuals who come to us seeking answers to significant health challenges. We use a few drops of a zinc solution and have the patient swirl it in their mouth for several seconds, then ask them what they tasted. The typical answer is "water," while the answer I am looking for is actually "metal," or a bitter taste.

As the clinical evidence continues, these same patients typically have a low enzyme in a blood serum comprehensive metabolic panel called **alkaline phosphatase**. The usual reference range for alkaline phosphatase in an adult is between 40 and 120. Ideally, I like to see the number be around 80. Historically, those with chronic health challenges may have a level of 45 or less. Just this one marker of deficiency in their body, determined either by blood serum, hair testing, and/or the taste test, may be their primary cause of poor health, including memory loss, depression, and anxiety. The exciting part, at least for me, is convincing someone they should cut back or eliminate completely the products containing wheat and soy.

Not having enough zinc would be like your grandmother, assuming she cooks, not having one essential ingredient for a favorite recipe. This is very important: one cofactor deficiency can compromise your health. Whoever would have thought a lack of vitamin C was the central fact causing thousands to die of a mysterious condition between 1750 and 1850 called scurvy? (I want to refer you back to the omega-3 metabolic fat chart, Chart #3 on page 11.)

> One cofactor deficiency can compromise your health.

If you look at Zn (zinc), it is necessary for the production of DHA via the Alpha-linolenic pathway (ALA). The pathway is a system where the body creates long-chain fats from the food you eat. I would suggest adding pumpkin seeds to your diet and minimizing wheat and soy. You will want to consider having your alkaline phosphatase checked and order the Aqueous Zinc from druglessdoctor.com and complete the Zinc Taste Test, or consider a Mineral Tissue Hair Analysis.

Aluminum & Memory Loss

Many years ago, aluminum was suspected as a factor for Alzheimer's, but that correlation has not provided a foundational hold. As a side note, I observed elevated aluminum levels on the Mineral Tissue Hair Analysis when the sodium and potassium levels were low, markers for adrenal fatigue or exhaustion. I am not suggesting aluminum is a factor in memory loss, but I want to point out the accumulation of toxic metals can occur when the adrenal glands are fatigued. We are regularly exposed to toxins. One way to help is to use chlorella, along with an adrenal support protocol, to help minimize heavy and trace toxic metal exposure.

Plaques & Memory Loss

The hypothesis, which appears to be holding up the longest when it comes to memory health, is the fact **tangles**, or plaques, are occurring in areas of the brain where the synapses (junctions where nerve fibers meet) are being compromised. There are many factors leading to memory deficiencies.

This is going to be a bit technical, but here is the key information you need to know about plaques. The plaques are described as amyloid beta

(Aβ) peptides, which are links of thirty-six to forty-three amino acids (protein building blocks) and are often involved with Alzheimer's. The links, or peptides, are the main components of the plaques found in the brains of Alzheimer's patients.[3] The best example I can think of for you is to imagine a big, thick spider web—the kind you see outside knotted up in a corner.

It has also been suggested the plaquing mechanisms may compete with insulin receptors in the brain. They may alter the energy-producing portion of cellular function. There is a massive amount of discussion regarding this topic.

Another view is that the plaques slow down, interrupt, and/or stop the information from transmitting from one nerve to the next. This is located at the synapse, or junction between nerves. Those promoting this viewpoint discuss a list of popular items contributing to plaque formation. From their perspective, this includes processed meats such as bacon, smoked turkey from the deli counter, and ham. Smoked meats like these contain nitrosamines, which cause the liver to produce fats that are toxic to the brain.

Here, I want to refer you back to the "Inside Out: Emotion" chapter (see Chapter Four). Your liver is associated with anger and is a significant player in the optimal function of fat metabolism, as well as clearing toxins from the body. I have noticed this more in individuals who have large livers while reviewing the results of standing digital radiographs. The liver may not be pathological (diseased) with abnormal serum enzymes increased from liver cell breakdown, but it can grow in size to satisfy the demand being placed on it from attempting to process food choices including sweet fruits, alcohol, and medications.

If you recall, my mom had an enlarged liver. She did not drink alcohol, but she ate a lot of sugar and fruit, a contributing factor for fatty livers. You want the liver to return to a normal size for optimal function. I have many patients who, by avoiding sugar, reducing fruit, and limiting the amount of "juice," notice a reduction in liver size. I have seen the liver reduce in size within three to six months, but keep in mind, it depends on the state of your liver health on how long it will take to see results.

Scientists have already recognized that exercise engages these receptors, and physical activity can slow the progression of Alzheimer's disease.

Amyloid, or the protein folding part of the plaque buildup on the brain, is found in Alzheimer's patients' brains. Amyloid may also cause inflammation on the brain's nerve cells. Again, I must emphasize inflammation is an epidemic today. Take a minute to look at your forearm and wrist. Now, look at your lower arm. Squeeze it. You should feel skin and then bone. If you feel a layer of fluid or "bogginess," you may think it is fat but it is your body holding onto water to keep pollutants in solution. You can be a thin person and still have this inflammation buildup in your body. You would just look a bit puffy.

If you can see and feel the fluid in your wrists, guess what? You are having the same squeezing of tissue in your brain and other areas of your body. There is only so much space available inside your skull, so something has to compensate. Don't let it be your brain's health!

Vitamin D & Memory Loss

Vitamin D and omega-3 fats can help decrease the plaque levels in people with Alzheimer's. A partial pilot[4] study published in the *Journal of Alzheimer's Disease* has indicated vitamin D3 and omega-3 fatty acids may support the immune system of the human body to reduce amyloid plaque levels.

It has also been suggested by scientists that Alzheimer's is not a result of abnormal production of the plaque. Instead, it is a result of impaired Aβ clearance or removal. The team discussing the subject suggested that anti-inflammatory protocols, including **cannabis-derived cannabinoids**, assist the plaque in crossing the blood-brain barrier. Cannabis, at the cellular level, is anti-inflammatory. I have seen in my practice those using CBD oils do experience temporary relief of joint pain. I personally am not sure if CBD oils will sustain an individual long-term unless they reduce inflammatory-based foods: sugar, fruit, dairy, red meat, and grains. The process of plaque-clearing is normal and fully functions for mentally active, healthy people. Prior materials suggest the clearing process is blocked in Alzheimer's patients.

What triggered my personal studies of memory research, amongst others, was the fact that vitamin D and omega-3 fats are two catalysts in the answer to helping those with memory loss. I believe it would be a wise choice to have your vitamin D levels and omega fats checked in order to determine your levels and then supplement according to the results.

Let's once again revisit my family's lifestyles. My mom exercised daily and dealt with memory loss. On the other hand, my mother-in-law ate fast food with deli meats filled with nitrates, and did not have a real or perceived plaque memory loss issue. She also did not like exercise. Knowing this insight, it comes down to the fact that I am not 100% sure if anyone knows the real cause. Taking the information that we do know and utilizing the protocol for your body, I know there will be a change.

Medications & Mental Health

I have been a proponent of reframing the effects of prescribed medications to all drugs have "bad effects," not just side effects. The words "side effects" feels expected and safe. The word puzzle and advertising game established by the prescription drug industry is deceiving as they mix and mince words. The most common of which is heartburn drugs, which create significant collateral harm and an assortment of side effects. All you have to do is listen to the drug advertisements throughout the media landscape. First, there are so many individuals who have digestive distress because they do not have enough digestive enzymes in their stomachs to begin with—just the opposite of what they are told. (Remember when I said brain health can be traced to your gut's health?)

> All you have to do is listen to the drug advertisements throughout the media landscape.

Your body utilizes B vitamins (yang) and minerals to create digestive enzymes. Sugar and stress deplete our systems of both B vitamins and minerals. If you do not have enough digestive secretions in your stomach, the food partially digests resulting in fermentation if it is a carbohydrate, putrefaction if it is a protein, and rancidity if it is fat. The "compost" pile in your stomach then creates excessive undesirable acids from the inappropriate process of "combustion," and hence, you have acid indigestion.

I mentioned earlier about the nervous system's impact on digestion. The nervous system controls and manages metabolism, while the brain sends signals and directions via the nerves and hormonal chemical transmitters. I have been personally trained and practice clinically as a nervous system healthcare provider through hands-on chiropractic care, which means I focus on the connection between the brain cells to tissue cells via spinal correction.

Chiropractic medicine is more than just neck and back pain. It is about the nervous system, which controls function regardless of what you may have been taught. The medical model is about an outside-in approach versus inside-out healing. At our practice we like to utilize the body's ability to heal itself. For example, if the brain is not able to communicate with the stomach because one of several nerve pathways is not up to par, you will have some distress. It is not uncommon for us to have a patient, who initially comes in with digestive distress as a secondary concern, ask us what we are doing while utilizing spinal correction because their digestive distress improves.

I can recall one young man tell me that he would take a digestive calcium aid every night before he went to bed. He realized it had been three months and the bottle was still full (where he used to go through a bottle a month). If you are contending with chronic digestive distress, you may consider adding the services of an experienced and well-skilled chiropractor who takes digital radiographs of your spine prior to starting your care. You are also welcome to visit our practices in Westlake, Ohio and Naples, Florida.

I recently had a sixty-eight-year-old patient concerned because she was told she had osteoporosis. They wanted to put her on either an injectable medication or an oral product to combat the bone breakdown. It is not uncommon for child-bearing women to have a long list of health challenges, including osteoporosis, which can be directly linked to carrying and having children.

Pregnant women have a greater demand placed on their livers while their child is developing in utero. Their livers are working overtime during the gestation period, which is supporting both the mother and the child. Having multiple children (in her case, five) created a common metabolic breakdown. Her liver was maxed out, burdened with clearing toxins and debris, and without the chance to go back to the pre-baby state. Her liver was not clearing estrogen, which resulted in uterine fibroids. Fibroids appear when there is excessive estrogen. The fibroids resulted in the removal of her uterus—while this procedure was being performed, they also removed her gallbladder.

> Pregnant women have a greater demand placed on their livers while their child is developing in utero.

Over time, she developed extreme digestive distress, so her medical team prescribed commonly used acid blockers, including Prevacid, Prilosec OTC, and Nexium. These medications interrupt the absorption of needed nutrients for mental health, memory, and bone health. The prescribed medications are now causing other problems, including an increased risk of Alzheimer's and dementia.

If you or someone you know has a history of digestive distress and/or they have had their gallbladder removed, it would be wise to add a digestive enzyme during their meals. Those with gallbladder removal would be wise to read the "Gallbladder Chapter" in my *Dr. Bob's Guide to Prevent Surgery.*

B12 Deficiencies & Memory

These same popular drugs for heartburn may lead to deficiencies in vitamin B12—a nutrient critical for brain and nervous system health. People who use these particular drugs for two years or more may have an increased risk of low vitamin B12 levels. This could lead to dementia and other severe symptoms. Vitamin B12 deficiency is relatively common, especially among older adults and those who primarily eat a plant-based diet. The number of those choosing the plant-only lifestyle is multiplying, which can and will result in our current millennials and future generations having a full-blown memory lapse epidemic.

Vitamin B12 deficiency has potentially severe medical complications when it goes undiscovered and/or undiagnosed. If left untreated, a vitamin B12 deficiency can lead to dementia, neurologic damage, anemia, and other complications, which may be irreversible. (This information appeared in the *Journal of the American Medical Association*[5] and recently, it was posted in *The Wall Street Journal.*)

Discovering the correlation between digestive distresses compounded by inappropriate medication protocols are essential to understand. As many as four in ten Americans have symptoms of acid reflux, and many depend on such drugs to control symptoms. This puts them at risk of a vitamin B12 deficiency. The problem may be particularly acute in seniors, who classically have a harder time absorbing the vitamin than younger patients. We see the impact of a deficiency in vitamin B12 at our practice.

In a recent study, doctors at Kaiser Permanente in Oakland, CA, looked at almost twenty-six thousand patients who had been newly diagnosed with a vitamin B12 deficiency. Those taking proton pump inhibitors, which alter stomach acid and nutrient absorption, and those taking another drug called H2RA, or a medication blocking histamine, had a B12 deficiency.[6] [7]

The higher the dose of acid-suppressing drugs someone is taking, the higher the risk of vitamin B12 deficiency. The link to a lack of vitamin B12 decreased after people stopped taking the drugs.

"At a minimum, the use of these medications identifies a population at higher risk of B12 deficiency, independent of additional risk factors," the author's wrote. "These findings do not recommend acid suppression for persons with clear indications for treatment, but clinicians should exercise appropriate vigilance when prescribing these medications and use the lowest possible effective dose." The researchers encourage patients who are taking or considering taking acid reflux drugs to discuss the risks and benefits with their doctors.

Other studies have shown that B12 and other B vitamins may be useful for the brain and help to keep memory sharp as one ages. It has been noted supplements of three B vitamins (folic acid, vitamin B6, and vitamin B12), appear to help to keep brain areas healthy. B vitamins are important for memory and one's mental capacity. This is important for the health of seniors with mild cognitive impairment, a form of memory loss, which can lead to Alzheimer's. Another study found B12 supplements can help to prevent brain shrinkage, a sign of possible Alzheimer's, and reduced brain function.

You can find vitamin B12 in meat and seafood. After age fifty, some individuals have trouble absorbing B vitamins from foods, particularly vitamin B12, and supplements are recommended. Those taking acid-suppressing drugs long-term will want to stay particularly vigilant in having their doctors monitor their B12 levels to help stave off possible memory problems and other symptoms like anemia and neurological problems.

Vitamin B12 is not easy to test. Clinicians routinely rely on the inexpensive serum B12 test, which measures the vitamin level in the blood. But this screening is not only unreliable, it is problematic for other reasons, including a lack of established cutoff points to define deficiency. From my experience, most individuals who have the test done have levels way past normal, which is not always validated by other correlations we have used.

In our practice, we observe several areas on a serum blood test. One of the markers we use for B12 levels includes the uric acid number. If it is low, we will support our patients with a sublingual B12 where the nutrient is absorbed directly into the system much the same way nitroglycerin helps one with chest pain. We also look at a group of blood markers found in a test called the CBC with differential. We look at the **MCV** (mean corpuscular volume), the **MCH** (mean corpuscular hemoglobin), and the **MCHC** (mean corpuscular hemoglobin concentration). Frequently, we will see these numbers at the higher levels of the reference range. There is also the Organix™ Urine Test that we incorporate, using a twenty-four-hour urine sample. If methylmalonate is increased in either of these samples, it can indicate a need for vitamin B12. People often have a difficulty with thinking about the time and task involved with this, but the results could be the answer they may be looking for.

Those markers suggest to us the patient has large, poorly oxygenated red blood cells, which in essence would suggest the brain is not getting its share of oxygen. Now, the challenge is that many wait until they are so far "gone" with low B12 that the sublingual product is not enough and B12 shots need to be administered.

I have witnessed those deficient in vitamin B12 become lethargic, unmotivated, tired, and unhappy. It does not necessarily have to be someone over the age of sixty-five. A red blood cell has about a 120-day cycle, so it will take time to see results, but it does make a difference. We look at the serum liver enzyme markers, AST and ALT, for vitamin B6 deficiencies. If they are low, we incorporate a **phosphorylated B6**, which is easier to absorb. There are several standard body signals for a B vitamin deficiency: crying without reason, sore muscles after exercise, noise sensitivity (raw nerves), a natural attraction of mosquitoes, and low blood pressure.

I have noticed that most women at about age forty begin to have digestive deficiencies, which actually can result in soft tissue pain, especially those who drink orange or grapefruit juice. We do not promote citrus, since the final result of its metabolism is an alkaline digestive state and essential mineral absorption is compromised. Also, we do not support alkaline water, which when used over time, can also interrupt healthy digestion. I encourage our patients to use minimal amounts of water when they eat, since water dilutes the pH in the stomach. Do not drink cold water with your meals, since this also disrupts the flow of blood to the entire digestive system.

Part of our overall problem is that physicians prescribe medications without a concrete follow-up plan.

On top of all of this, senior citizens who are in the US today are taking too many medications! It has been reported that 36% of those over age sixty-five take five or more medications per day. My patients tell me their primary care physicians cannot understand how they are getting along so well without drugs. So, part of our overall problem is that physicians prescribe medications without a concrete follow-up plan. As an individual, you need to take more responsibility for what you are taking, and ask questions of your providers and pharmacists.[7]

Helpful Reminders

- Journal your food and beverage intake. How much sugar are you consuming? This impacts vital cofactors for DHA production, which is needed for optimal brain and nervous system function.

- Consider the Zinc Taste Test. Standard zinc deficiency body signals include: large facial pores, white spots on your nails, your body heals "slowly," and wounds tend to scar easily. Men may notice pain on the inside of their heels because of the compressed nerve referral precipitated by a swollen prostate gland.

- Consider our Omega Oils Serum Profile to evaluate your levels of omega-3 and omega-6 fats, which will reveal if you have an abundance of inflammatory, omega-6 fats and arachidonic acid.

- A Mineral Tissue Hair Analysis will tell you if you have enough zinc, too much aluminum, and adrenal fatigue, plus many other significant findings.

- An Opti-Chem Profile will provide you with a series of answers, including if you have a vitamin B6 need, which can be evaluated with the lowered liver enzymes AST and/or ALT. A deficient B1 level is associated with reduced carbon dioxide (CO_2). The CBC with differential will clarify if you need B12. Vitamin B12 may also be considered deficient if you have decreased uric acid levels.

- A digestive aid with enzymes and digestive acids may support your digestion versus a proton pump inhibitor (PPIs).

Chapter Glossary

All definitions were sourced from the *Merriam-Webster Dictionary* unless otherwise noted.

Alkaline Phosphatase—Any of the phosphatases that are optimally active in alkaline medium and occur in especially high concentrations in bone, the liver, the kidneys, and the placenta

Amyloid—A waxy translucent substance consisting primarily of protein that is deposited in some animal organs and tissues under abnormal conditions (such as Alzheimer's disease)

Autonomic Nervous System—A part of the vertebrate nervous system that innervates smooth and cardiac muscle and glandular tissues and governs involuntary actions (such as secretion and peristalsis) and that consists of the sympathetic nervous system and the parasympathetic nervous system.

Central Nervous System—The part of the nervous system which in vertebrates consists of the brain and spinal cord, to which sensory impulses are transmitted and from which motor impulses pass out, and which coordinates the activity of the entire nervous system

Dementia—A usually progressive condition (such as Alzheimer's disease) marked by the development of multiple cognitive deficits (such as memory impairment, aphasia, and the inability to plan and initiate complex behavior)

Enteric Nervous System—One of the main divisions of the autonomic nervous system (ANS) and consists of a mesh-like system of neurons that governs the function of the gastrointestinal tract. (Wikipedia)

MCH (Mean Corpuscular Hemoglobin)—The number of grams of hemoglobin per unit volume and usually 100 milliliters of packed red blood cells that is found by multiplying the number of grams of hemoglobin per unit volume of the original blood sample of whole blood by 100 and dividing by the hematocrit

MCHC (Mean Corpuscular Hemoglobin Concentration)—The number of grams of hemoglobin per unit volume and usually 100 milliliters of packed red blood cells that is found by multiplying the number of grams of hemoglobin per unit volume of the original blood sample of whole blood by 100 and dividing by the hematocrit

MCV (Mean Corpuscular Volume)—The volume of the average red blood cell in a given blood sample that is found by multiplying the hematocrit by 10 and dividing by the estimated number of red blood cells

Notes

(1)   WHO; *Wall Street Journal,* Wednesday, May 15, 2019. Page A9. U.S. News.

(2)   "High Dose Zinc Supplementation Induces Hippocampal Zinc Deficiency and Memory Impairment with Inhibition of BDNF Signaling." https://www.ncbi.nlm.nih.gov/pmc/articles/PMC3561272/. Yang Yang, Xiao-Peng Jing, Shou-Peng Zhang, Run-Xia Gu, Fang-Xu Tang, Xiu-Lian Wang, Yan Xiong, Mei Qiu, Xu-Ying Sun, Dan Ke, Jian-Zhi Wang, and Rong Li.

(3)   Hamley, IW. "The Amyloid Beta Peptide: A Chemist's Perspective. Role in Alzheimer's and Fibrillization". Chemical Reviews, 112 (10): 5147–92, Oct 2012. doi:10.1021/cr3000994. PMID 22813427.

(4)   Champeau R. "Vitamin D, omega-3 may help clear amyloid plaques found in Alzheimer's." UCLA Newsroom, Feb 2013.

(5)   By www.ALZinfo.org, The Alzheimer's Information Site. Reviewed by William J. Netzer, Ph.D., Fisher Center for Alzheimer's Research Foundation at The Rockefeller University. MEDICATIONS

(6)   Lam, Jameson R., MPH; Jennifer L. Schneider, MPH; Wei Zhao, MPH; Douglas A. Corley, MD, Ph.D.: "Proton Pump Inhibitor and Histamine 2 Receptor Antagonist Use and Vitamin B12 Deficiency." JAMA, Vol 310, No. 22, December 11, 2013. MEDICATIONS

(7)   Too many older Americans take five or more medications. It's time to cut back: Olaoluwa Fayanju (Opinion) https://www.cleveland.com/opinion/2019/03/too-many-older-americans-take-five-or-more-medications-its-time-to-cut-back-olaoluwa-fayanju-opinion.html

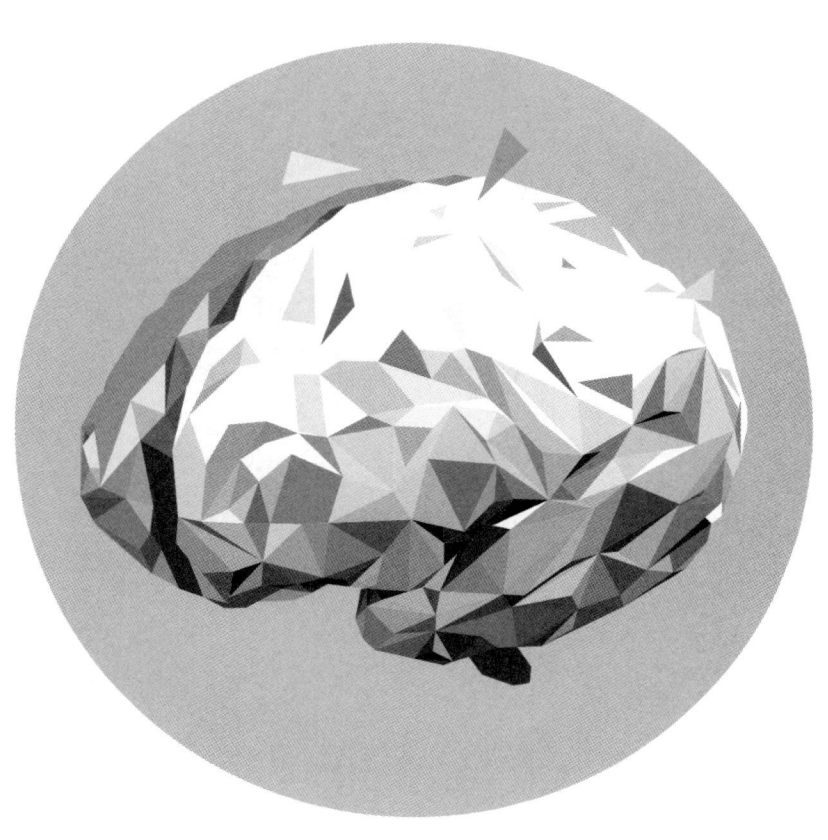

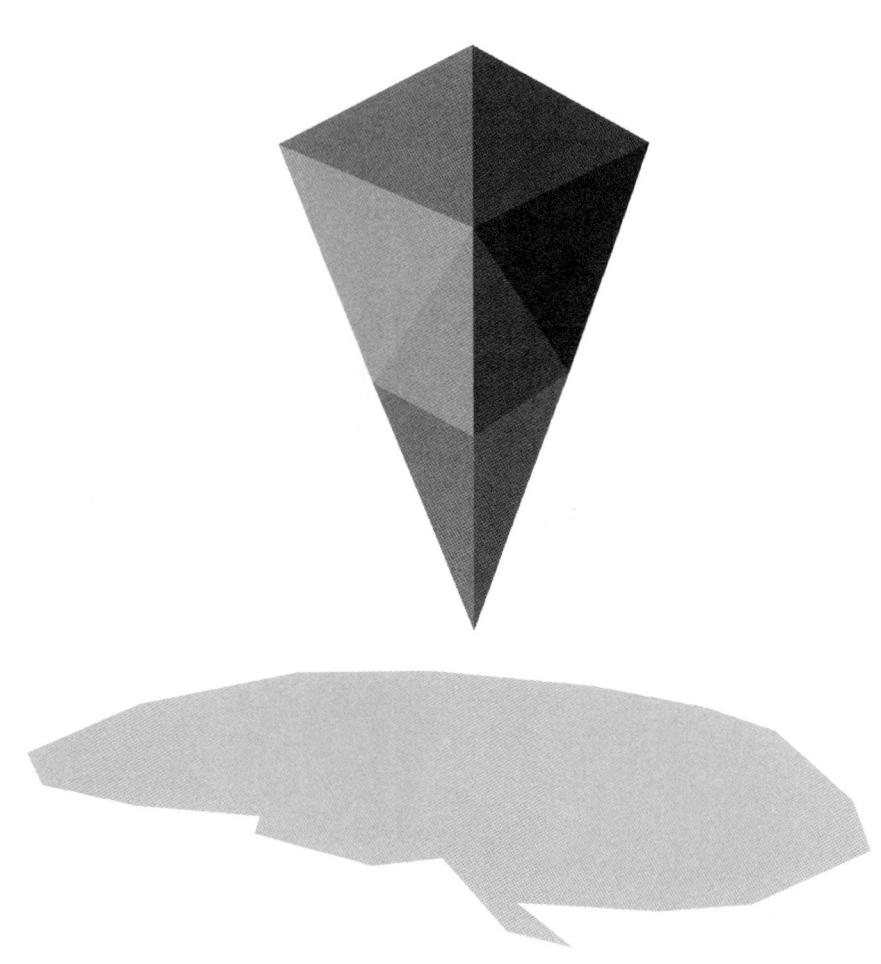

Chapter 7:

"WHERE DO I GO FROM HERE?": Mental Health Roadmap

If you're committed to helping improve your mental health naturally, you may be wondering, "Where do I begin?" The best answer is: Start with this chapter. Here you'll find recommended laboratory tests and nutritional support to lay a firm foundation on your path to recovery and freedom.

Prior to launching into this chapter, I feel a need to point out in one's mental health there is not one *specific* course of action which is the be-all end-all. There are some modalities and markers I have seen that can be used as a stepping-stone for everyone. With that said, let's begin!

My drugless mental health roadmap is one which focuses on creating a plan to establish normal levels of the omega oils which are needed to support optimal brain and nervous system function, whether the oil comes directly sourced from a marine product or is plant-based.

Step One: Mental Health-Friendly Nutrition

Omega-3 Oil: 1000mg before bed in order to establish an appropriate level of omega-3 oils.

- ▧ **Multiple Minerals: Supports the cofactors to create proper brain fat.**
- ▧ **L-Tyrosine: A natural antidepressant and constituent of thyroid hormone.**

- **5-Hydroxy Tryptophan:** A component creating adequate serotonin levels.
- **Vitamin B12:** Supports proper nervous system tissue.

The proper nutritional protocol would also include the cofactors or ingredients needed to create long-chain fatty acids for brain health via the plant-based alpha-linolenic pathway. Those ingredients would be determined by a comprehensive metabolic panel, in this case, an Opti-Chem Profile. The patient's vitamin B6, magnesium, and zinc levels can be determined and supplemented accordingly. The three cofactors are depleted with a stressful environment and sugar consumption.

Step Two: Omega-Oils Evaluation

The very first level to evaluate on a patient with any sort of mental health challenge would be the ratio of the omega-3 to omega-6 fats. Omega-3 oils are the brain-healthy oils used by the body to reduce inflammation and to support nervous system tissue.

Once a patient has completed the Omega Oils Serum Profile, the appropriate oils would be recommended. Now, in a situation where there may be an abundance of omega-6 to omega-3 oils causing inflammation and an increase in the byproduct of omega-6 surplus as in arachidonic acid, suggested recommendations would include avoiding sunflower and safflower oils. These omega-6 oils are used in abundance today in snack foods and restaurants. The abundance of omega-6 consumption will first increase the amount of linoleic acid. When noticed in excess, it suggests a substantial intake of those particular oils.

Supplementing with omega-3 oils alone is not enough in most cases; snack foods and especially the fats found in said foods and prepared products must also be reduced.

Evaluate the amount of EPA, which is the long-chain heart health fat, and DHA, the long-chain fat necessary for optimal brain and nervous system function. Low DHA is a factor suggesting a long-term nervous system fat deficiency.

Next, balance the omega-3 and omega-6 levels at a 1:1 ratio.

These omega-6 oils are used in abundance today in snack foods and restaurants.

- Evaluate using an Omega Oils Serum Profile, review the following levels: linoleic acid, arachidonic acid, EPA, and DHA. If there is excessive linoleic acid, you must read ingredient labels and stay away from sunflower and safflower oils. If the DHA is low, supplement accordingly, depending on the deficiency. At least 1000mg of an omega-3 anchovy and sardine-based oil should be consumed when the DHA levels are low.

- Evaluate the results of a comprehensive metabolic panel. The following levels should be assessed and treated accordingly; these are all needed to make brain-healthy fats from a plant source. Alkaline phosphatase levels should be at eighty and any amount less than this would suggest a zinc deficiency. The ALT and AST levels should be at least one-half of the total amounts in the lab's reference range. Low levels of these enzymes suggest a need for vitamin B6. The GTTP enzyme level, when low, suggests a need for magnesium and/or subpar thyroid function. Depending on the results, all three can be supplemented, or just those which are deficient. A zinc deficiency is common with those having memory challenges.

A proper amount of tyrosine is the most important step to securing long-term mental health stability. In severe situations, an Organix™ Urine Test is important to evaluate a variety of metabolites found in one's urine. One of the metabolites is VMA, which when in excess, suggests a high turnover of adrenal hormones and a potential to have low levels of amino acids, such as tyrosine. Tyrosine is a natural occurring antidepressant used by the body to make thyroid hormone when combined with iodine. A Thyroid Panel can also be completed to evaluate TSH, T3, and T4 levels. A low T4 may also suggest a need for tyrosine. If someone is depressed, and not taking an antidepressant, I would suggest they start on tyrosine. This can be initiated along with omega-3 oil, if indicated by the Omega Oils Serum Profile. Like I mentioned before, this would be my beginning protocol for a drugless approach to mental health concerns.

> A proper amount of tyrosine is the most important step to securing long-term mental health stability.

Step Three: 5-HIA & 5-HTP

Another metabolite of urine metabolism is 5-HIA, which when elevated, strongly suggests a high turnover of the brain neurotransmitter, serotonin. 5-HTP is an excellent nutrient, being a source of another protein building block called tryptophan. Tryptophan is used by the body to create serotonin; the primary purpose of most antidepressants is to selectively reabsorb serotonin. It would not be wise to supplement with 5-HTP if you are also taking a prescribed medication called an SSRI, or select serotonin reuptake inhibitor.

Step Four: Organix™ Urine Test

In this step, I would recommend an Organix™ Urine Test to evaluate your tyrosine and 5-HIA levels. If there is a high turnover of either of these metabolites, you would want to supplement with both tyrosine and serotonin, especially if you are not taking any medications. If you are not in a position to have your urine tested, it is ok to supplement with these products, but I would suggest you may want a minimum of the TSH, T3, and T4 levels.

Step Five: Determine Your Vitamin B Levels

The next step for most individuals would be to fill out a health assessment survey on page 74 to evaluate body functions and determine if you have the body signals of a vitamin B need. I discussed in Chapter Six the two types of B vitamins based on Traditional Chinese Medicine. Oftentimes, someone can be deficient in a B vitamin, resulting in "raw nerves." Common deficiencies of vitamin B would include: crying easily, sore muscles after exercise, waking up after sleeping for only an hour or two, low blood pressure, and if you are someone who mosquitoes find themselves attracted to. Your body needs B vitamins for optimal nervous system function. I have seen patient's mental challenges decrease by adding B vitamins to their supplement regimen. Keep in mind that sugar does deplete vitamin B from your body. Available in the Opti-Chem Profile.

Keep in mind that sugar does deplete vitamin B from your body.

Step Six: Vitamin B12 Lab Test

A final step in this protocol for an individual with mental stress and memory issues, who has a history of digestive distress and/or is currently taking a digestive drug, is a vitamin B12 test. I use a few determinants if someone does indeed require additional B12. The first would be to add a sublingual B12 product. Next, I look at the blood test called a CBC with differential. If the MCV or MCH and MCHC are elevated, you may need to supplement with vitamin B12. If and when you evaluate all of the B12 tests and you do not get a response or a change in the numbers, you may need to get B12 shots. Available in the Opti-Chem Profile.

All of the labs discussed in this chapter are available on druglessdoctor. com. Please use code MENTALHEALTH2020 to save 10% on your order.

Thank you!

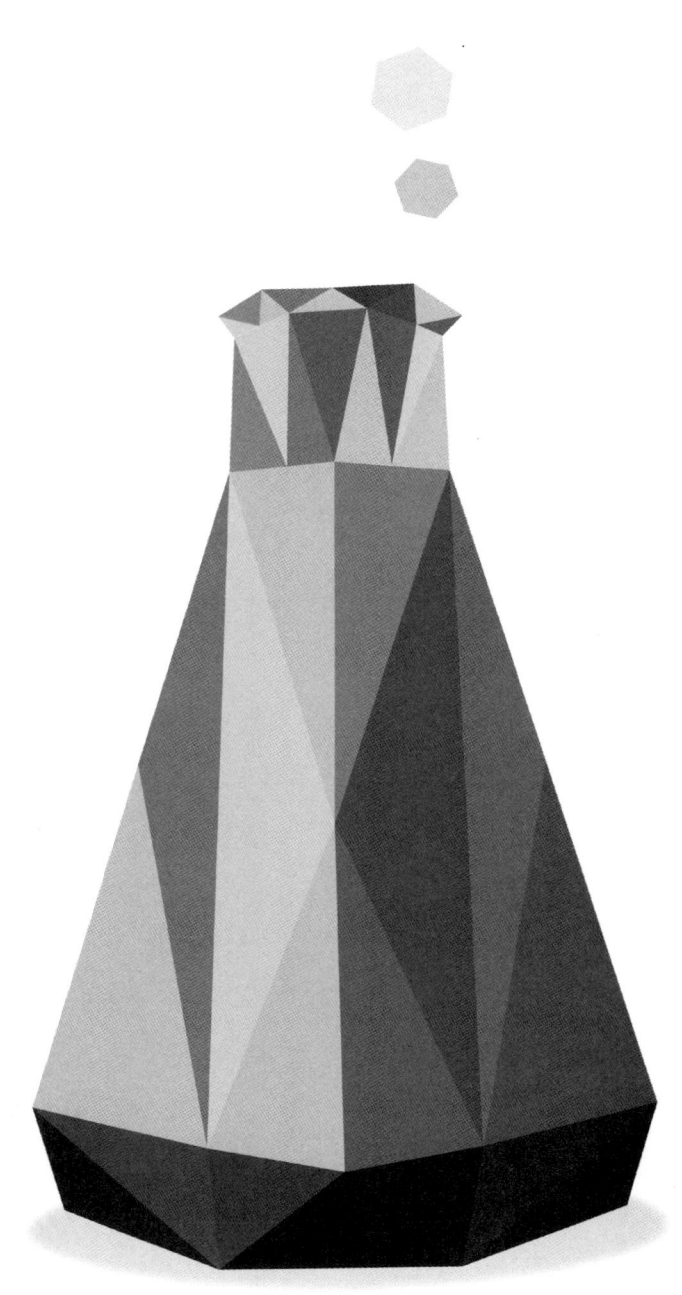

Chapter 8:

DRUGLESS LAB TESTING FOR OPTIMAL MENTAL HEALTH

When helping patients, we never "guess" about the protocol in which we personally create for them. One such way is through lab testing through trusted partners in order to provide accurate findings. We have helped many individuals who have come from other healthcare providers, either a Western-trained or a functional medicine practitioner, that do not provide a plan or post-test consultation. On the other hand, you may have left another healthcare professional's office with a bag of supplements without knowing what to do. I have witnessed both as our team of doctors and myself corrects and picks up the pieces of failed programs.

I have patients from all over the world who have had tests done and spent thousands of dollars at institutions without answers. I also connect with patients whose physicians do not know what to do with findings and literally just pass the results off. Side note: just the other day, we had one of our patients share with us that one of their friends was visiting a doctor who was searching the computer for answers to the patient's concern, when the actual answer should have been common knowledge for the physician.

I want you to be aware that properly prescribed medication (almost an oxymoron) by a well-meaning healthcare provider can actually be the reason why you may be having altered brain health, or any health-related condition for that matter. The most notorious drug of all is the proton-pump inhibitor (PPIs), or the "acid sopper" digestive drug. When you have gastric distress and start taking that medication, which neutralizes all acids, you potentially sabotage your body's ability to absorb useful nutrients and even end up worse than before you began.

Case in point, one female patient was on her PPIs for twenty years. Her serum alkaline phosphatase (see Chapter Six) was very low, which from a functional point of view, suggests a zinc deficiency. In previous chapters, you learned from me that zinc is a significant factor for optimal function. Zinc plays a vital role in metabolism of fat, skin, and memory. Her physician blamed her for the low alkaline phosphatase, explaining that she needed to drink more water. Now's the time to take control of your health! It may be an investment of finances and time in the beginning but will provide a healthier future for you and your family.

Now's the time to take control of your health!

> ## Online Lab Testing Available at druglessdoctor.com

Omega Oils Serum Profile

This test is an accurate tool to evaluate the amount of omega-3 and omega-6 fats in your body, along with linoleic and arachidonic acids. Omega-3 fats are necessary for optimal brain function, while on the other hand, omega-6 fats, when consumed in excess, create a state of inflammation. Linoleic acid is directly sourced from the omega-6 fats, which include sunflower, safflower, soybean, canola, and corn oils. When these oils are a primary staple in your diet, they will be transported to another "backup" metabolism. Eating omega-6 fats for a long period of time can result in a diversion of those inflammatory oils to pathways which includes arachidonic acid (pain producing and inflammatory). Any serious health plan to prevent Alzheimer's should include the Omega Oils Serum Profile.

Opti-Chem Profile

The Opti-Chem Profile is a combination of specific tests we have created to use in our practice, which consists of: fasting glucose, uric acid (low with a vitamin B12 deficiency), BUN, creatinine, sodium, potassium, chloride, C02, magnesium, calcium, phosphorous, total protein, albumin, globulin, LDH, bilirubin, alkaline phosphatase (low with a zinc deficiency), ALT,

AST, GTTP, and serum iron. The findings from this panel significantly help determine the potential for optimal function.

CBC with Differential (Included in the Opti-Chem Profile)

The complete blood count (CBC) with differential offers many insights into one's health puzzle. With this assessment and reading its results, one can correlate causes, including a chronic infection (bacterial vs. viral). We also look at markers that may suggest a vitamin B12 need, food sensitivities, gut health concerns, and parasites. Oxygen is carried by blood, and if the markers for the red blood cells are abnormal, the results should be treated to enhance oxygen transport. Through this test, I have discovered many individuals can have aspirin-induced anemia. This is a unique challenge and is common today because many people from all over the world take their "baby" aspirin pill daily. Aspirin can deplete the body of blood over time. Many usually do not give a thought to the bleeding potential, which means, there is less blood to carry oxygen to the brain.

Thyroid Testing

Thyroid Serum Panel

The thyroid tests we offer display how well your thyroid gland is working. Your thyroid gland is the gas pedal of the body and has everything to do with the speed of your metabolism. Individuals with weight problems, depression, brain fog, anxiety, and constipation often have impaired thyroid function. Our Thyroid Serum Panel provides information about how well your brain is sensing various thyroid hormone levels. Furthermore, these tests show how your immune system is interacting with your thyroid, and if you are under stress.

One key takeaway for understanding the thyroid is that your pituitary gland located in your brain creates a hormone called thyroid stimulating hormone (TSH). The thyroid gland, when stimulated, is designed to create T4, which is the inactive form of thyroid hormone, which converts to T3 (the active form). If the T4 to T3 conversion is impaired, I usually suspect there is a stressful situation creating a deficiency of cofactors which we support through our thyroid protocols.

To screen for problems, most conventional doctors test only for TSH. I have had patients tell me that some of their providers blatantly refuse to order other thyroid markers. However, as T3 is one of the body's master molecules, it is important to know your T3 levels. For example, T3 helps regulate digestion, energy use, and hormonal balance. Still, it is possible the physicians only know what to do with a patient when their TSH is high because they are limited in their prescription drug selection and very few individuals even recognize there is a need for iodine. Also, the primary, or go-to medication, they have to prescribe for thyroid function only has T4.

> Lifestyle factors, especially nutrition (avoid gluten), are essential for long-term optimal health and healing.

On the other hand, we use a neonatal porcine glandular product along with iodine, optimal EFAs, and zinc (if the lab results indicate a need) for those with only a subpar thyroid. This is the first step to help one's thyroid have nuclear components, with elevated TSH to help the patients begin to feel better. Of importance, lifestyle factors, especially nutrition (avoid gluten), are essential for long-term optimal health and healing.

Serum TPO Test

An autoimmune disease called Hashimoto's thyroiditis is a common self-seeking and destroy response often associated with hypothyroidism. We have created a protocol combining vitamin E and selenium with an elimination of gluten to help reduce the response.

To screen for thyroid autoimmunity, I order a panel to measure thyroid peroxidase antibodies (TPO). This is what I have learned about the optimal levels of thyroid function from my forty plus years of experience.

If someone has adrenal gland fatigue, depression, and low blood pressure, which drops even lower from a sit to a stand position, I may also recommend an Organix™ Urine Test to evaluate if there is a tyrosine deficiency. Determining a tyrosine need can go a long way to supporting thyroid gland function, the creation of adrenal hormones, and a brain hormone called dopamine.

We use a diversified approach to assess the entire body. If a female has breast or ovarian cysts, or a man has an enlarged prostate, we may consider a Urine Iodine Loading Test and/or a Serum Iodine. Iodine is necessary for a variety of functions, including apoptosis—programmed cell death that keeps cancer cells in check.

Vitamin B12 Test

Adequate levels of vitamin B12 are critical for brain health, yet nearly 40% of Americans are deficient in this vitamin. Gut dysbiosis, poor digestion (often from hypothyroidism), eating inflammatory foods, and using acid sopper medication can cause a B12 deficiency. Specifically, heartburn medication suppresses stomach acid and blocks the absorption of vitamin B12.

Vitamin B12 can be considered as an important antidepressant factor, and is essential in making red blood cells, line nerve cells, and keeps our brains functioning properly. A B12 deficiency has been linked to deep depression, paranoia, and memory loss. Furthermore, pregnant women who are deficient in vitamin B12 may put their babies at risk for neurological disorders, developmental delays, and cognitive and motor impairments. It's important to note that blood tests for B12 don't share with you the entire story. This vitamin works inside cells, and blood levels won't tell you your brain levels of B12. Therefore, it's helpful to complement this test by measuring homocysteine.

Homocysteine is an inflammatory protein that is metabolized by vitamin B12 and folate. When someone has high blood levels of homocysteine, it indicates that vitamin B12 is low. This surrogate marker provides more information on how well your brain and body are functioning.

I also like to look at serum uric acid levels (Opti-Chem Profile), that when low, suggest a need for B12. Also, vitamin B12 is important for the size, amount, and concentration of iron in a red blood cell. We order a CBC with differential in our standard protocol. If the differential has elevated levels of MCH, MCHC, and MCV, it may suggest a need for B12. We also look at the liver enzymes AST and ALT; when low, they suggest a vitamin B6 need, which helps coordinate MCH and MCHC levels.

C-Reactive Protein

C-reactive protein (CRP) is another general marker of inflammation. Numerous studies, including meta-analysis, have analyzed tens of thousands of people and show that elevated CRP is associated with depression and anxiety.

Fasting Glucose, Insulin, and Hemoglobin A1C

These tests check blood sugar control. The most noteworthy of these tests is Hemoglobin A1C, as it gives an average of your blood sugar levels over the past 90 to 120 days. The fasting glucose test provides a snapshot of how much sugar is present when your body isn't processing food properly. The fasting insulin test gives insight on how your pancreas is functioning while you're not eating.

Mineral Tissue Hair Analysis

We use the Mineral Tissue Hair Analysis to evaluate a variety of metabolic systems including digestion, adrenal, and thyroid health. Using the ratios assists us in the evaluation of metabolic activity. Zinc levels, for example, can be low in comparison to copper, which may in fact be elevated, creating an imbalanced ratio. High copper levels are common with a diet primarily focused on grains and soy. There are many markers to glean from this test in order to create a proper mental health protocol.

Organix™ Urine Test

The Organix™ Urine Test is an efficient tool to evaluate the metabolites of function in the body. There are a variety of markers that can either be elevated and/or deficient, which when analyzed, help solve the puzzle regarding all aspects of one's health, including mental stability.

Helpful Reminders

- All of the labs discussed in this chapter are available on druglessdoctor. com. Please use code MENTALHEALTH2020 to save 10% on your order.

- The Omega Oils Serum Profile and Opti-Chem Profile are the two tests we recommend as the foundation towards a drugless mental health plan.

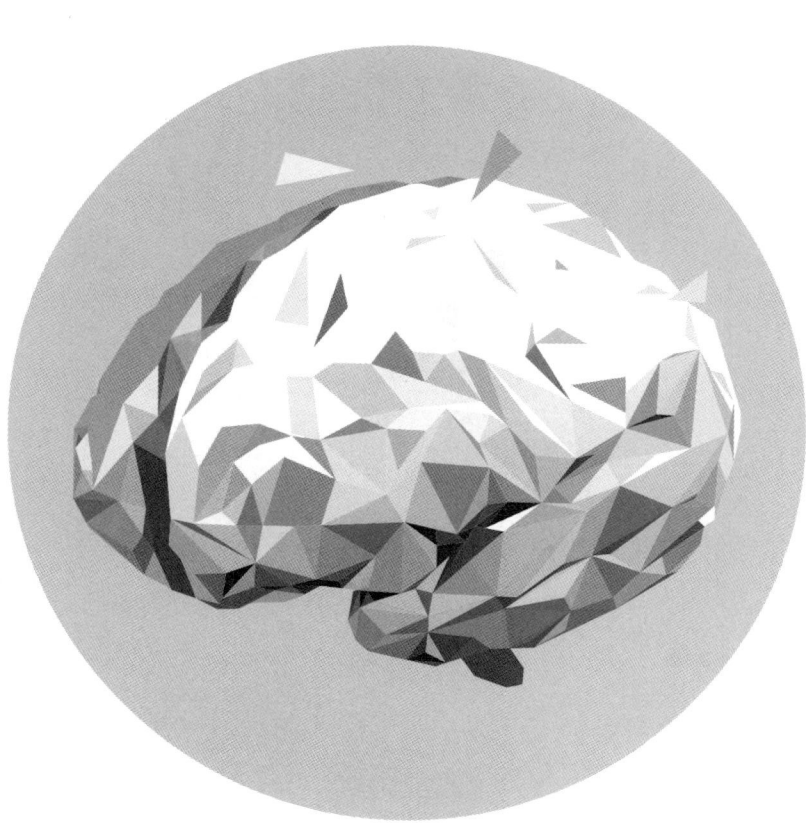

Appendix A:
21 HABITS TO HELP YOUR MENTAL HEALTH

Why twenty-one? It's been said that it takes twenty-one days to begin a habit, and we have put together a tangible list that you can begin today. These have worked for me and I know they will work for you!

1. Begin your day with gratitude. If you are someone who prays, that is always a great way to start!

2. Once a month, journal what you are thankful for.

3. Ask yourself: How can I help someone today?

4. Write a letter to a friend or family member. I can't tell you how good it feels to receive a letter from a friend in the mail.

5. Volunteer your time. Find a local non-profit and commit to helping once a month.

6. Take ten deep breaths throughout the day.

7. Do a crossword puzzle to help stimulate your brain and memory.

8. Have an accountability partner to share how you are really feeling.

9. Write forgiveness letters to those who you need to forgive. Once you're done, read them out loud, then rip them up and throw them away. I know you will feel better.

10. Have an honest monthly conversation with yourself. Share what emotions you experienced throughout the past month and how you handled situations that may have affected you in some way.

11. Make sure to move in some sort of capacity each day, yes, this means exercise. Find something you enjoy, whether it is walking, tennis, mountain biking, or ping pong.

12. Take time to rest. This looks different for each person, but whatever you can do to let your brain be at ease, do that! I give myself Sunday to recharge and be with family.

13. Watch what the lyrics really say when you're listening to music. I would never speak some of today's lyrics in my life. Call me crazy, but I know you'll notice a difference too!

14. Have a game night with friends. Break out games from your childhood and have a good laugh!

15. Print off pictures from your phone camera or regular camera and then post them where you can view the happy memories throughout the day.

16. Say "Please" and "Thank You" and other courtesies that it seems are being forgotten.

17. Hold the door open for those who are right behind you.

18. Do everything without complaining.

19. Only speak good and positive things about yourself.

20. Make a meal with friends without anyone posting a picture to social media.

21. End your day by giving it to God, and then going to sleep.

Appendix B:

ZINC TASTE TEST

Instructions

Place a small amount of **Aqueous Zinc**™ solution in the mouth (~10ml) and hold for thirty seconds. Describe your initial taste according to the following categories (for accurate results, refrain from eating, drinking or smoking for at least one half hour prior to the test).

Response 1: No specific taste or other sensation is noticed after the solution has been held in the mouth for up to thirty seconds.

Response 2: No immediate taste is noted, however, after a few seconds a slight taste develops, variously described as "dry," "mineral," "furry," or "sweet."

Response 3: Definite, though not a strongly unpleasant taste is noted almost immediately and tends to intensify with time.

Response 4: A strong unpleasant taste is noted almost immediately.

Key

Response 1: Strongly suggests zinc deficiency and favorable response to zinc supplementation.

Response 2: Suggests zinc deficiency and favorable response to zinc supplementation.

Response 3: Suggests zinc is likely inadequate with need for zinc supplementation.

Response 4: Suggests zinc is adequate with no need for zinc supplementation.

Zinc Facts

Zinc is essential to good health. Dozens of zinc dependent enzymes participate in a myriad of health defining metabolic functions. Classic signs of zinc deficiency include:

- **Severe Deficiency**—Delayed healing of ulcers, neurosensory disorders, infections due to immune dysfunction, weight loss, skin inflammation, baldness, diarrhea, sexual underdevelopment in males, and emotional disorders.

- **Moderate Deficiency**—Growth retardation, delayed wound healing, neurosensory changes, immune dysfunction, rough skin, poor appetite, mental lethargy and sexual underdevelopment in males.

- **Mild Deficiency**—Decreased muscle mass, neurosensory changes, inability to react, sluggishness, decreased immune system functions, and decreased sperm count and testosterone in males.

LIT-132 Rev. 12/08
© Copyright 2008

Appendix C:

THE CHEF'S GARDEN HOME DELIVERY

As I'm sure you can imagine, I have been able to visit many sources of sustainable farming throughout my career, but I have never tasted food that was so nutrient-dense, fresh, and "alive" as I have at The Chef's Garden.

Located in my neck of the woods in northern Ohio, The Chef's Garden grows specialty vegetables, microgreens, and herbs. They also are well-regarded in the hospitality industry and provide produce daily to many restaurants with Michelin stars.

Their success is born from the like-minded work and sustainable farming philosophies that they share with their customers, which is derived from a steadfast will to not only survive but thrive in agriculture. This commitment to delivering the highest quality, most nutritionally dense, flavorful, fresh vegetables, microgreens, herbs, edible flowers, and more direct from Earth-to-Table® and their willingness to listen carefully to a consumer's needs is what motivates and enriches their work and inspires them each and every day.

We are happy to offer the following optimal health vegetable boxes for home delivery:

- Visit https://www.chefs-garden.com/products/home-delivery.

- Select "Anti-Aging Mix," "Detoxification Mix," or "Optimal Health Mix."

- Currently the boxes are priced at ninety dollars and freight will be charged based on the shipping option chosen and the location of delivery.

- To order, you will need to create an account at this web address: https://www.chefs-garden.com/help/customer-service/create-an-account.

- If you would like to have a recurring order, please contact info@chefs-garden.com directly. They can get you set up.

As always, wishing you happiness and wellness,
Dr. Bob & Debbie

**Please be sure to add "Drugless Drs." in
the comments section at the end of the order.**

INDEX

About the Author

Dr. Bob DeMaria has been helping patients with natural, drugless care since the 1970s. Over his career, he has noticed a progressive decline in the quality of life of new patients coming into his office. The incidence of surgeries and invasive procedures has escalated to the point where nearly every new patient, young or old, has been prescribed a medication or has experienced some type of surgical intervention. These facts have motivated Dr. Bob to pursue natural, drugless answers for conditions that are occurring in epidemic proportions and continuing at an alarming rate. Hundreds of thousands of hysterectomies, cholecystectomies (gallbladder extractions), and other organ removals and surgeries can be prevented by making appropriate lifestyle modifications.

Dr. Bob has a bachelor's degree in human biology. He is a practicing D.C. (doctor of chiropractic) and has relentlessly continued with his post-graduate education, earning a natural health doctor (NHD) degree, fellow status in spinal engineering, and diplomat status in treating bone and joint conditions without medication. Dr. Bob graduated valedictorian of his class with honors. He is a recognized worldwide expert and is frequently a keynote speaker.

Dr. Bob teaches post-graduate-level, continuing-education classes in the health, business, legal, and teaching areas. He has been a college instructor, and has spoken in Europe and Canada. He has been on television internationally, and he hosts his own weekly regional TV program with his wife of over forty years, Deb. They have two sons.

Dr. Bob has ten other popular books focusing on natural health restoration: *Dr. Bob's Guide to Stop ADHD in 18 Days*, *Dr. Bob's Trans Fat Survival Guide*, *Dr. Bob's Guide to Optimal Health*, *Dr. Bob's Drugless Guide to Detoxification*, *Dr. Bob and Debbie's Guide to Sex and Romance*, *Dr. Bob's Men's Health—The Basics*, *Dr. Bob's 1 Minute a Day to a Healthier You*, *Dr. Bob's Drugless Guide to Balancing Female Hormones*, and *Dr. Bob's Guide to Prevent Surgery*, *Dr. Bob's Guide to a Healthy Marriage*. Like his other books, *Dr. Bob's Drugless Guide to Mental Health* is an accumulation of over forty years of experience that will surely help make a difference in anyone's life.

Dr. Bob knows it is time for the public to take control of their own future regarding the state of their personal health. He experiences that it can work: he sees it happen every day. The information in this book will make a difference. All you have to do is take action. Today is your day!

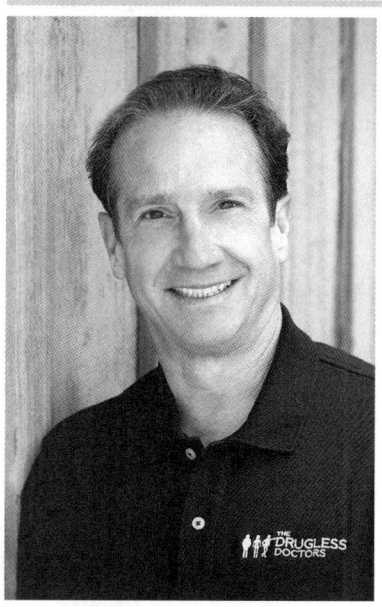

Dr.Bob
The Drugless Doctor

ONLINE CLASSES

We want to welcome you to our online classroom!

We're so excited to be starting this digital education journey, where Dr. Bob will serve as your personal guide in your pursuit towards optimal health.

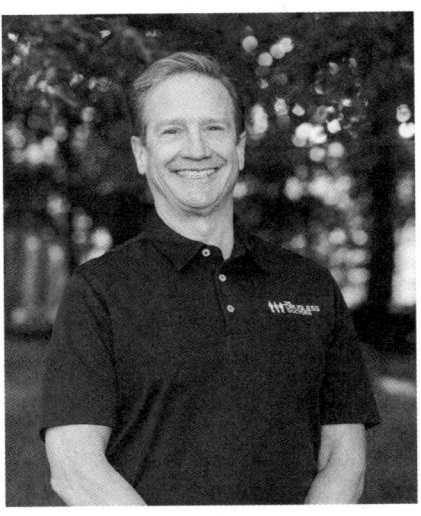

Based on clinical observations and forty-plus years of experience, each class is designed with you in mind to provide a clear roadmap to take charge of some of today's top health topics, including hormones, detoxification, stress, and mental health at a price that is affordable for everyone.

Once you have finished each class, you'll receive a certificate of completion, because we want to celebrate your achievements!

Are you ready to change your health and your life? Let's begin!

Learn More, classes.druglessdoctor.com

We are happy to partner with the YouVersion App with devotionals on topics on marriage, mental health, women's health, and more.

Dr.Bob
The Drugless Doctor

YouVersion

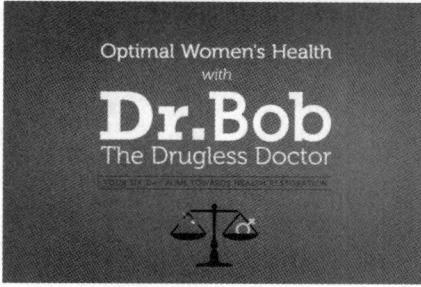

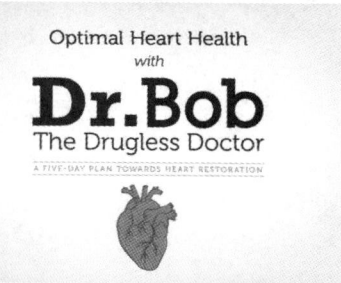

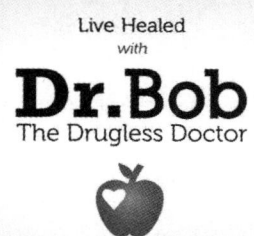

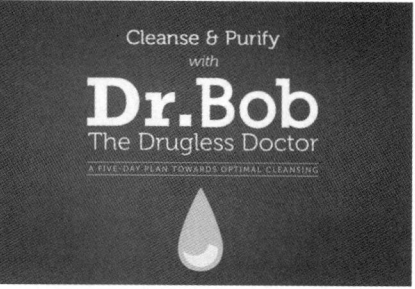

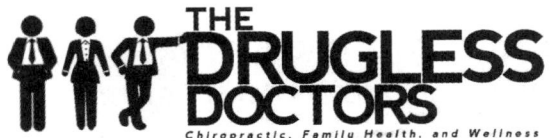

THE DRUGLESS DOCTORS

Chiropractic, Family Health, and Wellness

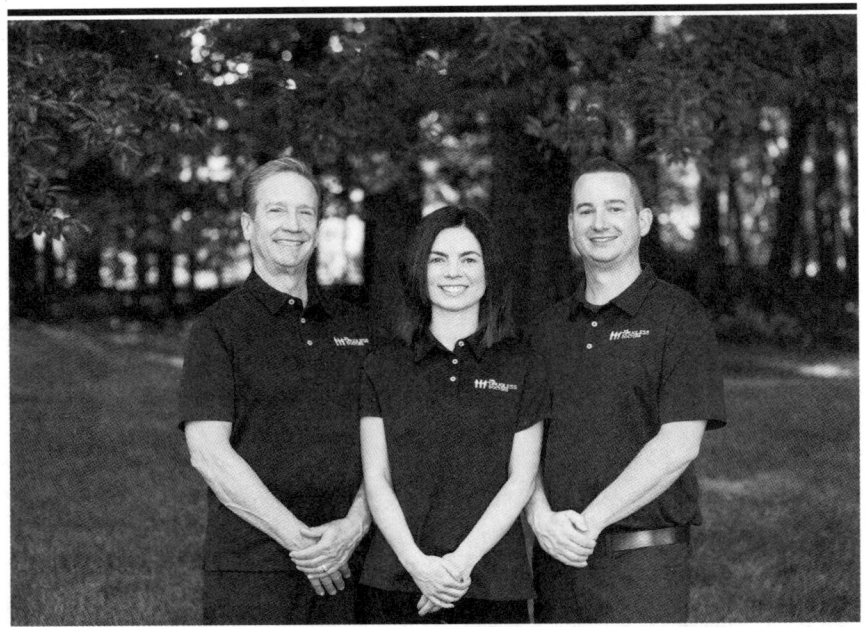

Dr. Bob, Dr. Casen, and Dr. Anthony

SPECIALIZATIONS INCLUDE:

- Motion Specific Chiropractic
- Pediatric Chiropractic
- Digital Fluoroscopy
- Breast Thermography and More